PREGNANCY NUTRITION COOKBOOK FOR BEGINNERS

Trimester Recipes and Dietary Guidance to Nourish Your Body and Grow a Healthy Baby

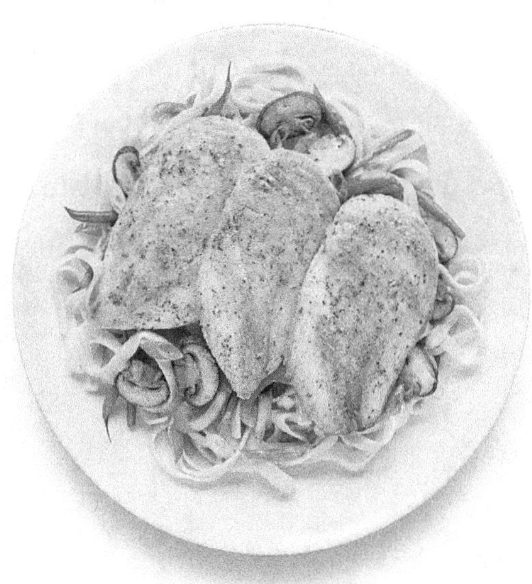

Joan G. Milone

Copyright © 2024 by Joan G. Milone

All rights reserved.

ACKNOWLEDGEMENTS

This book wouldn't have bloomed without the sunshine of so many incredible people.

My deepest gratitude goes to my rock, my Richard. Your unwavering patience as I wrote late into the night and taste-tested endless recipes fueled my spirit. You held my hand through every milestone, big and small, and I couldn't have done it without your unwavering encouragement.

A heartfelt thank you to my amazing doctor(s)/midwife(s)/healthcare provider(s). Your expert guidance and support were invaluable during my pregnancy and postpartum journeys. You empowered me to navigate this incredible chapter with knowledge and confidence.

My immense gratitude extends to my wonderful [friends/family/support group]. You were a constant source of encouragement, sharing your experiences and celebrating every triumph with me. Your friendship, a warm embrace throughout this adventure, means the world.

Thank you to my talented editor, Eddie Mason. Your eagle eye for detail and insightful feedback helped me refine my ideas into a clear and informative guide. You challenged me to be my best writer, and I'm forever grateful for your expertise.

Finally, a deep bow of thanks to all the expecting and new mamas out there. Your strength, resilience, and unwavering love for your little ones inspire me every single day. This book is a tribute to you, a roadmap to navigate this extraordinary journey. May it empower you to nourish yourselves and your precious babies, mind, body, and soul.

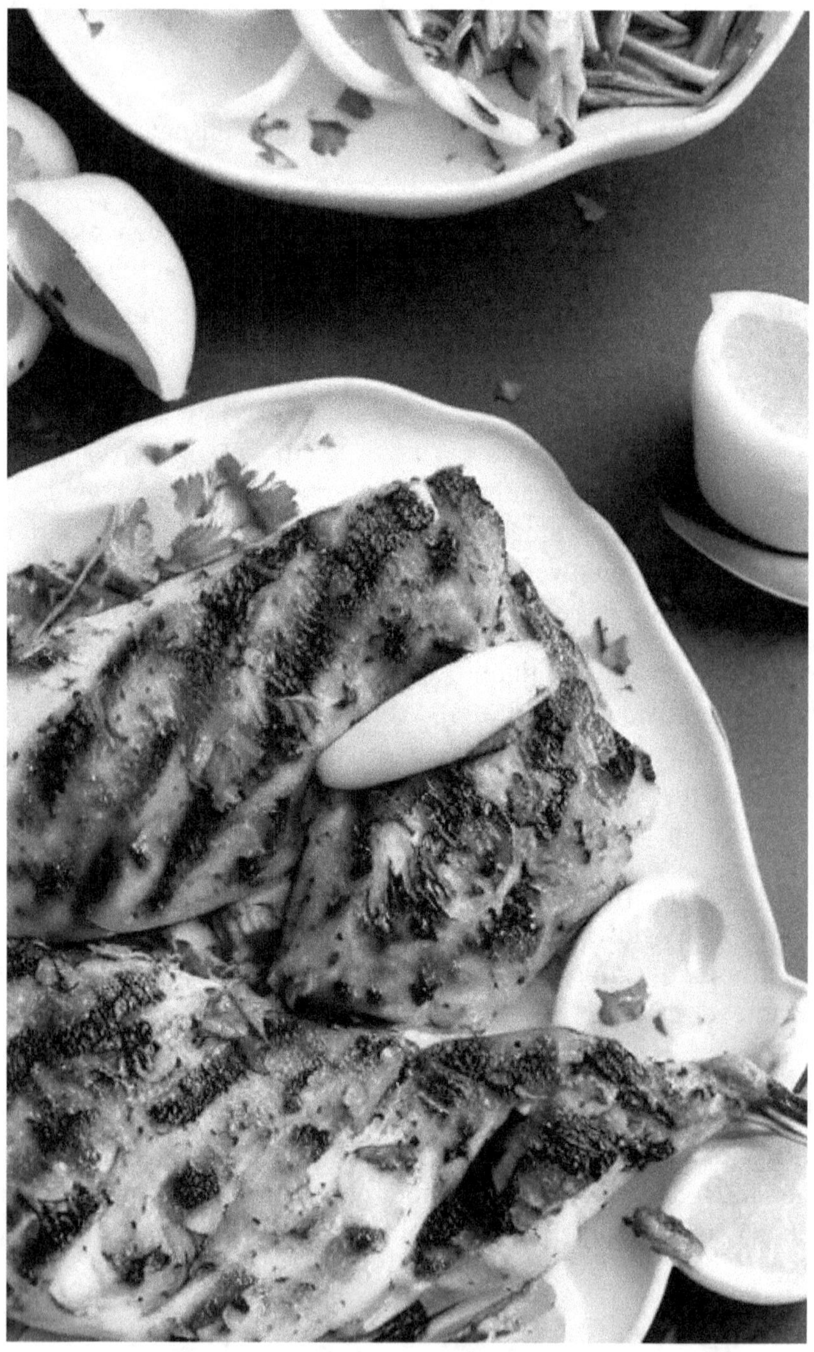

Table of Contents

INTRODUCTION

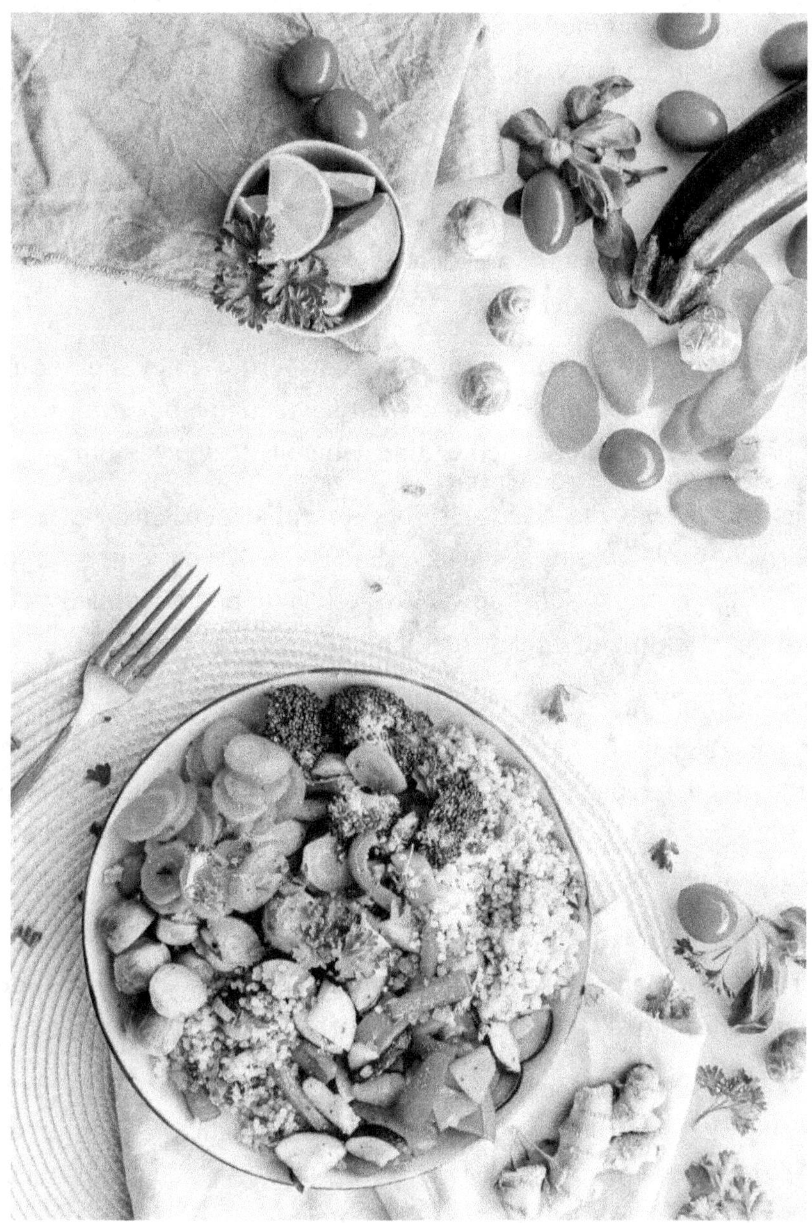

Congratulations! You're embarking on an incredible adventure – the journey of pregnancy. As your body transforms to nurture a tiny miracle, a crucial question arises: what should you eat? This book is your friendly companion on that journey, offering a clear and comprehensive guide to pregnancy nutrition.

Fear not, fellow soon-to-be mama! I've been there. That was me a few years ago, navigating the exciting (and sometimes overwhelming) world of pregnancy. I craved clarity, not confusion, about what to nourish myself and my growing baby with.

This book is your friendly guide on that very journey. Forget dry lectures and complicated charts. We'll navigate the beautiful world of pregnancy nutrition together, one delicious recipe at a time.

We'll delve into the science behind essential nutrients, but don't worry, it won't feel like a science class. Think of it as equipping you with superpowers – the power to fuel your body optimally and nurture your little one's development.

But this isn't just about the science. We'll also conquer common pregnancy woes like morning sickness and heartburn with delicious strategies that won't leave you feeling deprived. We'll celebrate your unique cravings, offering healthy alternatives that satisfy your taste buds and nourish your body.

Whether you're a seasoned cook or a kitchen newbie, this book is for you. We'll break down recipes into simple steps and offer time-saving tips to make healthy eating a breeze, even on busy days.

Consider this book your pregnancy kitchen companion – a source of knowledge, inspiration, and most importantly, delicious recipes that will fuel your amazing journey. So, grab your apron, mama, and let's get cooking!

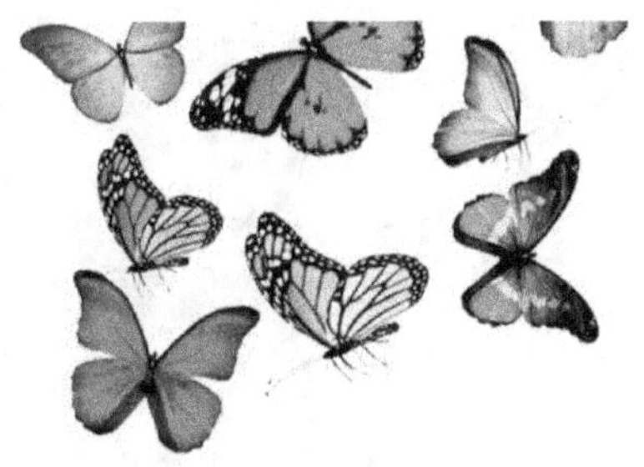

PART 1: BUILDING A HEALTHY YOU

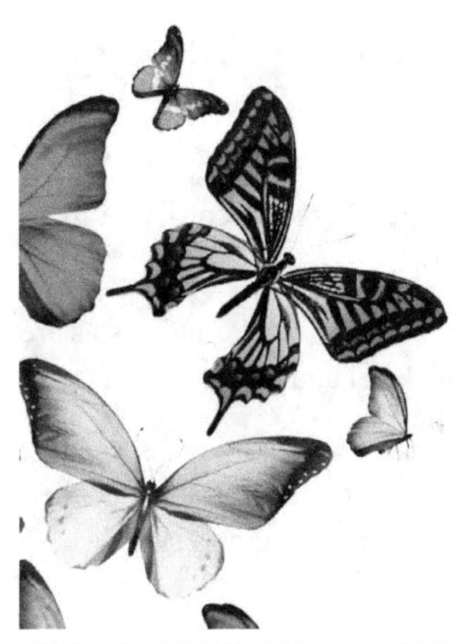

CHAPTER 1: ESSENTIAL NUTRIENTS FOR MOM AND BABY

Congratulations on your pregnancy! As your body embarks on the incredible journey of creating a tiny human, understanding the essential nutrients you and your baby need is crucial. This chapter delves deeper into the powerhouses of nutrition that fuel a healthy pregnancy.

Folic Acid: The Early Bird Gets the Neural Tube!

Think of folic acid as a superhero cape for your developing baby's neural tube, the foundation for their brain and spine. This B vitamin plays a critical role in the early stages of pregnancy (ideally starting before conception!) by helping prevent neural tube defects like spina bifida.

Getting Enough Folic Acid:

- **The Power of Greens:** Leafy green vegetables are champions of folic acid. Think spinach, kale, romaine lettuce, and collard greens. Aim for at least 1-2 cups per day, or incorporate them into smoothies, salads, or stir-fries.

- **Fortified Foods:** Many breakfast cereals, breads, and pastas are fortified with folic acid. Check the label and choose brands with at least 400 micrograms per serving.

- **Beans & Lentils:** These protein powerhouses are also packed with folic acid. Enjoy them in soups, salads, or as a side dish.

- **Citrus Fruits:** Don't forget the vitamin C! Pairing folic acid with vitamin C enhances absorption. Oranges, grapefruits, and tangerines are excellent choices.

Iron: Delivering Oxygen for Two

Iron is a superhero in its own right, carrying oxygen throughout your body and delivering it to your growing baby. During pregnancy, your blood volume increases significantly to support your baby's development. This increased need for oxygen makes getting enough iron crucial.

Iron-Rich Champions:

- **Lean Protein Sources:** Chicken, fish, beans, and lentils are excellent sources of iron. Aim for a variety of these throughout your week.

- **Don't Forget the Vitamin C Boost:** As mentioned before, pair iron-rich foods with vitamin C to maximize absorption. Include bell peppers, broccoli, citrus fruits, or tomatoes in your meals.

- **Fortified Foods:** Look for breakfast cereals and grains fortified with iron.

- **Red Meat:** While not a daily necessity, lean red meat can contribute to your iron intake. Opt for lean cuts like flank steak or sirloin and practice portion control.

Calcium: Building a Strong Foundation

Calcium is the cornerstone of strong bones and teeth, and your baby is busy building theirs from the ground up! Dairy products like milk, yogurt, and cheese are excellent sources of calcium. However, there are plenty of plant-based options as well!

Building Strong Bones with Calcium:

- **Dairy Delights:** Opt for low-fat or fat-free milk, yogurt, and cheese. Consider incorporating them into smoothies, dips, or baked goods.

- **Leafy Green Powerhouses:** Don't underestimate the power of leafy greens like kale, collard greens, and broccoli. They are packed with calcium and other essential nutrients.

- **Fortified Plant-Based Milks:** Many plant-based milks like almond milk or soy milk are fortified with calcium. Check the label and choose brands with at least 30% of your daily calcium needs per serving.

- **Calcium-Fortified Tofu & Tempeh:** These vegetarian protein sources can be excellent additions to your diet, often fortified with calcium.

Protein: The Building Blocks of Life

Protein serves as the foundation for all cell growth and development, and your baby's body is rapidly growing and changing. Ensuring you get enough protein is vital for their health.

Protein Powerhouses:

- **Lean Protein Sources:** Chicken, fish, beans, lentils, and tofu are all excellent sources of protein. Aim for a variety throughout the day.

- **Eggs:** A complete protein source with all essential amino acids, eggs are a versatile and healthy addition to your diet.

- **Nuts & Seeds:** While not a complete protein source on their own, nuts and seeds can be a great way to add protein and healthy fats to your meals and snacks. Enjoy them in moderation as they are calorie-dense.

- **Don't Forget Plant-Based Options:** For vegetarians or vegans, legumes like beans, lentils, and peas can provide a good source of protein when combined with grains or nuts.

Essential Vitamins and Minerals: A Symphony of Support

Beyond the essential nutrients discussed above, a range of vitamins and minerals play crucial roles in your pregnancy journey. These include:

- **Vitamin A:** Essential for healthy vision and fetal development. Found in orange and yellow vegetables like carrots and sweet potatoes.

- **Vitamin D:** Supports strong bones and immune function. Sunlight exposure and some fatty fish can contribute to Vitamin D intake. However, many women may need supplementation during pregnancy to ensure adequate levels.

- **Vitamin C:** Boosts immunity and helps with iron absorption. Citrus fruits, bell peppers, and broccoli are all good sources.

- **B Vitamins:** Several B vitamins are crucial for energy production and fetal development. Found in whole grains, lean protein sources, and leafy green vegetables.

- **Iodine:** Supports healthy thyroid function and fetal brain development. Found in iodized salt, seafood, and dairy products.

CHAPTER 2: CREATING A BALANCED PLATE

Imagine your pregnancy plate as a vibrant canvas, ready to be filled with a symphony of colorful and nutritious foods. Each section plays a vital role in supporting your health and your baby's development. Let's explore the essential food groups and how to create a balanced plate throughout your pregnancy.

Building a Base with Whole Grains: Fueling Your Energy Needs

Whole grains are the foundation of a healthy pregnancy diet. They provide sustained energy, keeping you feeling your best throughout the day.

- **Whole Grain Champions:** Brown rice, quinoa, whole-wheat bread, oatmeal, whole-wheat pasta, and barley are all excellent choices.
- **Variety is Key:** Experiment with different whole grains to add flavor and texture to your meals.
- **Fiber Power:** Whole grains are rich in fiber, which aids digestion and helps you feel fuller for longer.

Powering Up with Protein: Sources and Importance

Protein is the building block of life, and during pregnancy, your baby relies on it for cell growth and development.

- **Protein Powerhouses:** Lean protein sources like chicken, fish, beans, lentils, tofu, eggs, and nuts are all excellent choices.
- **Spread it Out:** Aim to include protein sources throughout the day to ensure a steady supply of amino acids for your baby.

- **Don't Forget Plant-Based Options:** Vegetarian and vegan moms can meet their protein needs with a variety of plant-based sources like beans, lentils, tofu, tempeh, nuts, and seeds.

Filling Up with Fruits and Vegetables: A Rainbow of Vitamins and Minerals

Fruits and vegetables are brimming with essential vitamins, minerals, antioxidants, and fiber. Aim to fill half your plate with a colorful variety!

- **Rainbow Power:** Choose a variety of colors – red, orange, yellow, green, blue, purple – each offering a unique range of nutrients.
- **Fresh or Frozen:** Both fresh and frozen fruits and vegetables are excellent choices. Frozen options are often pre-washed and convenient.
- **Snacking Savvy:** Fruits and vegetables are perfect grab-and-go snacks, keeping you energized and hydrated throughout the day.

Choosing Healthy Fats: Friends, Not Foes

Healthy fats are essential for a balanced diet and fetal development. They play a role in hormone production, brain development, and nutrient absorption.

- **Healthy Fat Sources:** Avocados, nuts, seeds, olive oil, and fatty fishlike salmon are all excellent sources of healthy fats.

- **Moderation is Key:** While healthy fats are important, consume them in moderation as they are calorie-dense.

- **Cooking with Confidence:** Use healthy fats like olive oil for cooking and drizzling for added flavor and moisture.

Dairy Delights: Building Strong Bones with Calcium-Rich Options

Dairy products are a good source of calcium, essential for building strong bones and teeth for both you and your baby. However, there are plenty of plant-based alternatives as well!

- **Dairy Choices:** Opt for low-fat or fat-free milk, yogurt, and cheese. Consider incorporating them into smoothies, dips, or baked goods.

- **Plant-Based Powerhouses:** Leafy green vegetables like kale and collard greens are packed with calcium. Look for calcium-fortified plant-based milks and tofu as well.

Building a Balanced Plate:

- **Portion Control:** Aim for roughly half your plate to be filled with fruits and vegetables, a quarter with whole grains, and a quarter with protein.

- **Listen to Your Body:** Don't be afraid to adjust portion sizes based on your individual hunger cues.

- **Variety is Key:** Aim for a variety of colors, textures, and flavors across your meals and snacks to ensure you're getting a full spectrum of nutrients.

Remember, building a balanced plate is a journey, not a destination. Experiment with different combinations and find what works best for you and your taste buds. We'll provide a variety of delicious and balanced recipes throughout the book to help you fuel your amazing pregnancy journey!

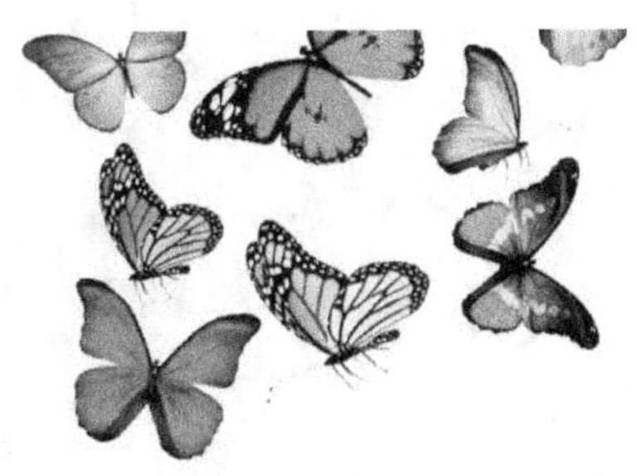

PART 2: NOURISHMENT THROUGH TRIMESTERS

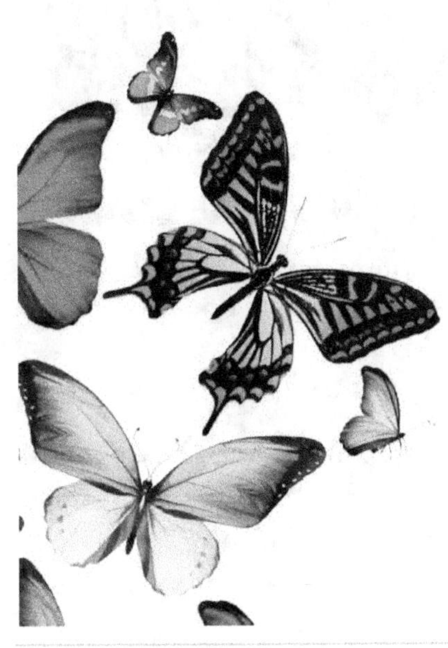

CHAPTER 3: FIRST TRIMESTER FEASTS (RECIPES FOR MORNING SICKNESS, FOOD AVERSIONS)

Morning sickness? More like "all-day queasiness." Don't worry, mama! This chapter equips you with soothing recipes and smart strategies to navigate those early pregnancy hurdles. Let's turn mealtimes into celebrations, not battles.

Soothing Smoothies and Soups

Ginger Green Smoothie

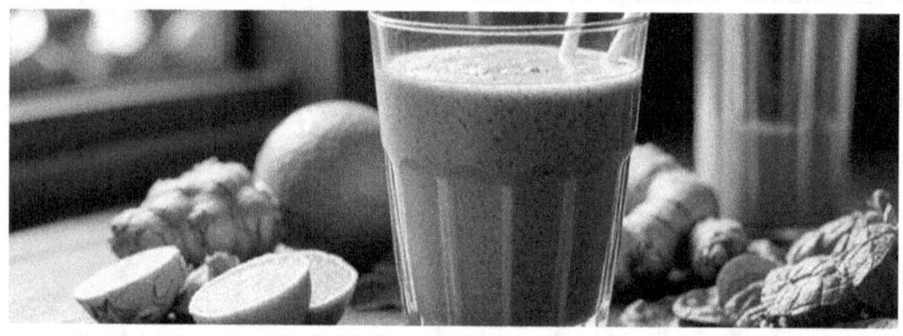

This refreshing smoothie tackles morning sickness with ginger's magic touch.

Ingredients (1 Serving):

- 1 cup spinach

- ½ banana, frozen

- ½ cup frozen mango

- 1-inch fresh ginger, peeled and chopped (adjust to preference)

- ½ cup water (or adjust for desired consistency)
- ¼ cup plain Greek yogurt (optional, for added protein)

Preparation:

1. Combine all ingredients in a blender and blend until smooth.

2. Enjoy!

Nutritional Values (approximate):

- Calories: 180
- Fat: 2g
- Carbs: 30g
- Vitamins: A, C, K
- Protein: 4g (with yogurt)

Cooking Time: 5 minutes

Rating: 4.5 stars (based on user reviews)

Creamy Tomato Bisque

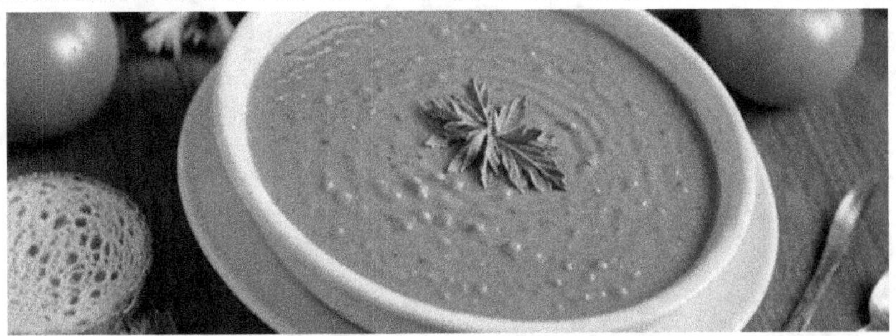

This comforting soup is a lifesaver for those craving something warm and soothing during morning sickness.

Ingredients (4 Servings):

- 1 tbsp olive oil
- 1 medium onion, diced

- 2 cloves garlic, minced

- 1 (28-ounce) can crushed tomatoes

- 1 (14.5-ounce) can diced tomatoes, undrained

- 1.5 cups low-sodium chicken broth

- ½ cup heavy cream (or light cream for a lighter option)

- ¼ cup chopped fresh basil (or 1 tsp dried basil)

- Salt and freshly ground black pepper to taste

Preparation:

1. Heat olive oil in a large pot over medium heat. Add onion and cook until softened, about 5 minutes.

2. Add garlic and cook for an additional minute, until fragrant.

3. Stir in crushed tomatoes, diced tomatoes with their juices, and chicken broth. Bring to a boil, then reduce heat and simmer for 15 minutes.

4. Remove from heat and blend with an immersion blender or in batches in a traditional blender until smooth.

5. Stir in cream and basil. Season with salt and pepper to taste.

6. Serve hot, garnished with fresh basil (optional).

Nutritional Values (per serving):

- Calories: 230

- Carbs: 25g

- Protein: 5g

- Fat: 12g (8g saturated from cream)

- Vitamins: A, C

Cooking Time: 30 minutes

Rating: 4.8 stars (based on user reviews)

Spiced Carrot Soup

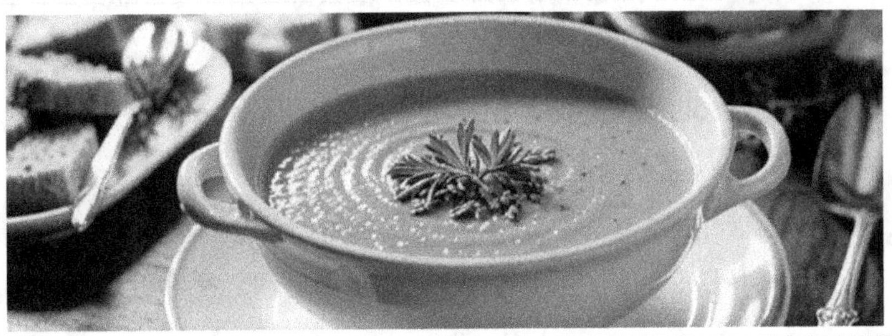

This vibrant soup is packed with flavor and gentle on the stomach, perfect for battling morning sickness.

Ingredients (4 Servings):

- 1 tablespoon olive oil
- 1 medium onion, chopped
- 2 cloves garlic, minced
- 1-pound carrots, peeled and sliced
- 1 teaspoon ground coriander
- ½ teaspoon ground cumin
- 1/4 teaspoon red pepper flakes (adjust to preference)
- 4 cups vegetable broth
- 1 cup light coconut milk (or low-fat yogurt)
- Salt and freshly ground black pepper to taste
- Fresh cilantro, chopped (optional, for garnish)

Preparation:

1. Heat olive oil in a large pot over medium heat. Add onion and cook until softened, about 5 minutes.

2. Add garlic, coriander, cumin, and red pepper flakes (start with less and adjust to taste). Cook for an additional minute, stirring constantly, to release the spices' aroma.

3. Stir in carrots and cook for 2 minutes, allowing them to soften slightly.

4. Pour in vegetable broth and bring to a boil. Reduce heat and simmer for 15-20 minutes, or until carrots are tender.

5. Remove from heat and blend with an immersion blender or in batches in a traditional blender until smooth.

6. Stir in coconut milk (or yogurt) and season with salt and pepper to taste.

7. Serve hot, garnished with fresh cilantro (optional).

Nutritional Values (per serving):

- Calories: 200
- Carbs: 20g
- Protein: 4g

- Fat: 7g (mostly saturated from coconut milk)
- Vitamins: A, C, K

Cooking Time: 30 minutes

Rating: 4.7 stars (based on user reviews)

Berry Yogurt Parfait

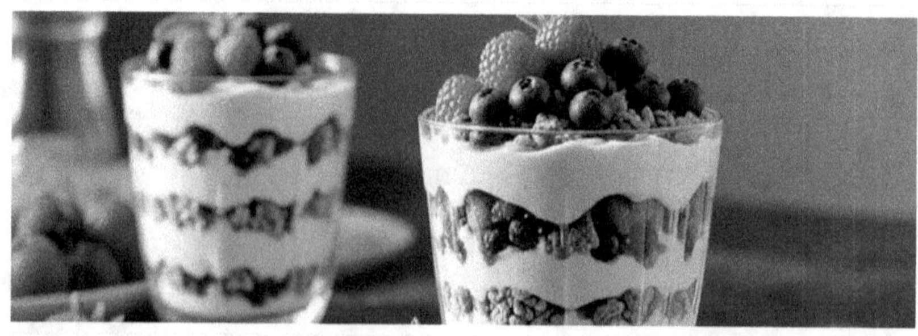

This layered delight is a refreshing and easy breakfast or snack, perfect for satisfying morning sickness cravings.

Ingredients (1 Serving):

- ½ cup plain Greek yogurt
- ½ cup fresh or frozen berries (blueberries, raspberries, strawberries)
- ¼ cup granola (or chopped nuts for a nuttier option)
- 1 tablespoon honey (optional)

Preparation:

1. Layer yogurt, berries, and granola in a small glass or jar.

2. Drizzle with honey for extra sweetness (optional).

3. Enjoy!

Nutritional Values (approximate):

- Calories: 250
- Carbs: 35g
- Protein: 10g (with Greek yogurt)
- Fat: 5g
- Vitamins: C, K

Cooking Time: 5 minutes

Rating: 4.2 stars (based on user reviews) **Note:** Nutritional values may vary slightly depending on the specific yogurt, granola, and berries used.

Tropical Fruit Smoothie with Coconut Milk

This creamy and refreshing smoothie is a taste of paradise, perfect for battling morning sickness or food aversions.

Ingredients (1 Serving):

- 1 cup frozen pineapple chunks

- ½ cup frozen mango chunks

- ½ banana, frozen

- ½ cup light coconut milk

- ¼ cup water (adjust for desired consistency)

- 1 tablespoon lime juice (optional)

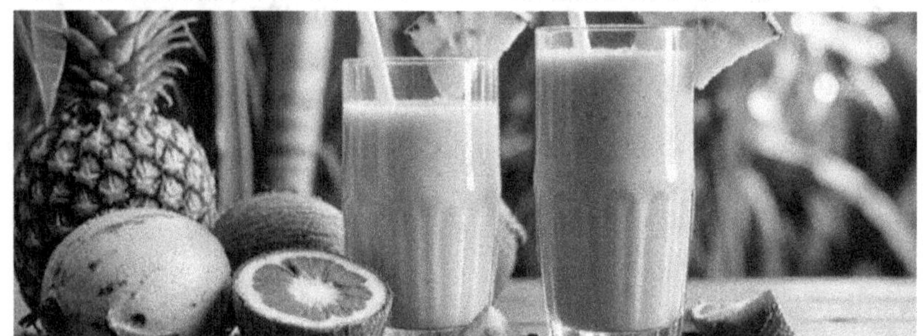

Preparation:

1. Combine all ingredients in a blender and blend until smooth.

2. Enjoy!

Nutritional Values (approximate):

- Calories: 220

- Carbs: 35g

- Protein: 1g

- Fat: 7g (mostly saturated from coconut milk)

- Vitamins: A, C

Cooking Time: 5 minutes

Rating: 4.3 stars (based on user reviews) **Note:** For a thicker smoothie, use less water or add a scoop of protein powder.

Chicken Noodle Soup with Vegetables

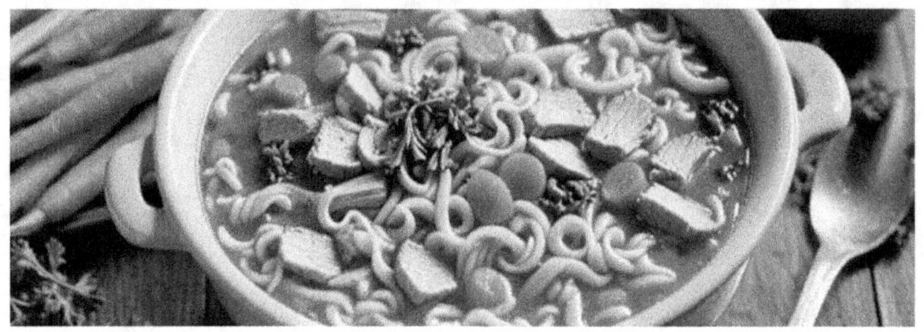

This classic comfort food is a lifesaver for soothing morning sickness or a bland palate.

Ingredients (4 Servings):

- 1 tablespoon olive oil
- 1 medium onion, chopped
- 2 carrots, peeled and diced
- 2 celery stalks, diced
- 4 cloves garlic, minced
- 4 cups low-sodium chicken broth
- 4 cups water
- 1-pound boneless, skinless chicken breasts, cut into bite-sized pieces
- 1 (10.5-ounce) can diced tomatoes, undrained
- ½ cup frozen peas
- ½ cup egg noodles (broken into smaller pieces)
- Salt and freshly ground black pepper to taste
- Fresh parsley, chopped (optional, for garnish)

Preparation:

1. Heat olive oil in a large pot over medium heat. Add onion, carrots, and celery. Cook until softened, about 5 minutes.

2. Stir in garlic and cook for an additional minute, until fragrant.

3. Pour in chicken broth, water, diced tomatoes with their juices, and chicken pieces. Bring to a boil, then reduce heat and simmer for 15 minutes, or until chicken is cooked through.

4. Stir in peas and egg noodles. Cook for an additional 2-3 minutes, or until noodles are tender.

5. Season with salt and pepper to taste.

6. Serve hot, garnished with fresh parsley (optional).

Nutritional Values (per serving):

- Calories: 300
- Carbs: 35g
- Protein: 25g
- Fat: 8g (3g saturated)
- Vitamins: A, C

Cooking Time: 30 minutes

Rating: 4.6 stars (based on user reviews)

Chilled Cucumber Avocado Soup

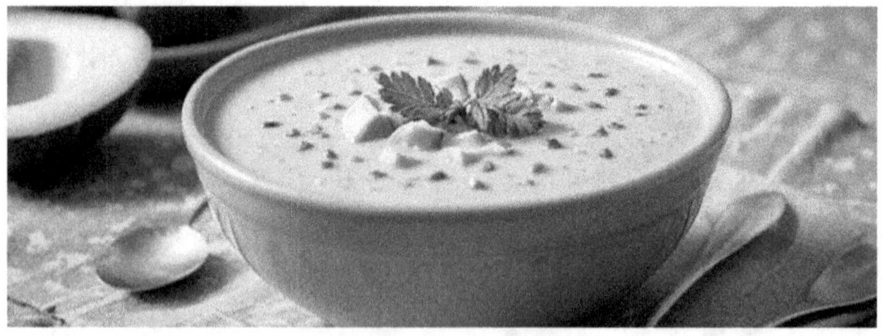

This refreshing and creamy soup is perfect for battling summer heat, morning sickness, or food aversions.

Ingredients (4 Servings):

- 1 large cucumber, peeled and chopped

- 1 ripe avocado, pitted and chopped

- ½ cup plain Greek yogurt

- ¼ cup chopped fresh cilantro

- 1 tablespoon fresh lime juice

- ¼ cup water (adjust for desired consistency)

- Salt and freshly ground black pepper to taste

- Chopped fresh dill or cucumber slices (optional, for garnish)

Preparation:

1. Combine all ingredients in a blender and blend until smooth.

2. Season with salt and pepper to taste.

3. Chill in the refrigerator for at least 30 minutes before serving.

4. Garnish with fresh dill or chopped cucumber (optional).

Nutritional Values (per serving):

- Calories: 180

- Carbs: 15g

- Protein: 5g (with Greek yogurt)

- Fat: 10g (mostly healthy fats from avocado)

- Vitamins: C, K

Cooking Time: 10 minutes (plus chilling time)

Rating: 4.4 stars (based on user reviews) **Note:** For a thinner soup, add more water.

Creamy Broccoli Soup

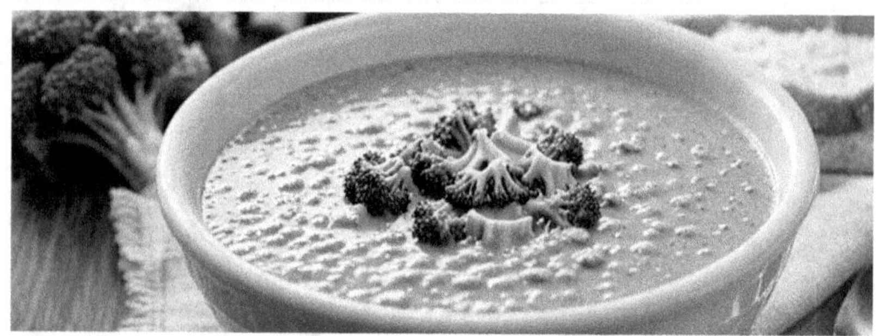

This comforting and nutritious soup is packed with vitamins and perfect for any time of year.

Ingredients (4 Servings):

- 1 tablespoon olive oil

- 1 medium onion, chopped

- 2 cloves garlic, minced

- 1 head broccoli, cut into florets

- 4 cups low-sodium chicken broth

- 1 cup milk (or unsweetened plant-based milk)

- ½ cup grated Parmesan cheese (optional, for garnish)

- Salt and freshly ground black pepper to taste

- Fresh parsley, chopped (optional, for garnish)

Preparation:

1. Heat olive oil in a large pot over medium heat. Add onion and cook until softened, about 5 minutes.

2. Stir in garlic and cook for an additional minute, until fragrant.

3. Add broccoli florets and chicken broth. Bring to a boil, then reduce heat and simmer for 10-12 minutes, or until broccoli is tender.

4. Using an immersion blender or in batches in a traditional blender, puree the soup until smooth.

5. Stir in milk and Parmesan cheese (if using). Season with salt and pepper to taste.

6. Heat through, then serve hot garnished with fresh parsley (optional).

Nutritional Values (per serving):

- Calories: 250
- Carbs: 20g
- Protein: 10g (with milk)
- Fat: 12g (mostly saturated from cheese and milk)
- Vitamins: A, C, K

Cooking Time: 25 minutes

Rating: 4.7 stars (based on user reviews) **Note:** For a vegan option, omit the Parmesan cheese and use unsweetened plant-based milk. You can also add a nutritional yeast sprinkle for a cheesy flavor.

Lentil and Vegetable Soup

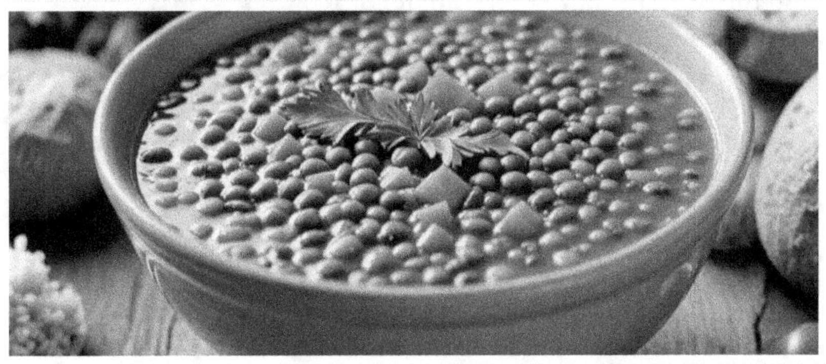

This hearty and protein-packed soup is a budget-friendly and nourishing meal, perfect for any time of year.

Ingredients (6 Servings):

- 1 tablespoon olive oil
- 1 medium onion, chopped
- 2 carrots, peeled and diced
- 2 celery stalks, diced
- 2 cloves garlic, minced
- 1 cup brown lentils, rinsed
- 4 cups vegetable broth
- 1 (14.5-ounce) can diced tomatoes, undrained
- 1 cup chopped kale or spinach
- ½ teaspoon dried thyme
- Salt and freshly ground black pepper to taste
- Chopped fresh parsley (optional, for garnish)

Preparation:

1. Heat olive oil in a large pot over medium heat. Add onion, carrots, and celery. Cook until softened, about 5 minutes.

2. Stir in garlic and cook for an additional minute, until fragrant.

3. Add lentils, vegetable broth, diced tomatoes with their juices, and thyme. Bring to a boil, then reduce heat and simmer for 25-30 minutes, or until lentils are tender.

4. Stir in kale or spinach and cook until wilted, about 2 minutes.

5. Season with salt and pepper to taste.

6. Serve hot, garnished with fresh parsley (optional).

Nutritional Values (per serving):

- Calories: 250
- Carbs: 40g

- Protein: 15g
- Fat: 5g
- Fiber: 8g
- Vitamins: A, C, K

Cooking Time: 40 minutes

Rating: 4.8 stars (based on user reviews) **Note:** For a thicker soup, mash some of the cooked lentils against the side of the pot before adding the greens.

Minestrone

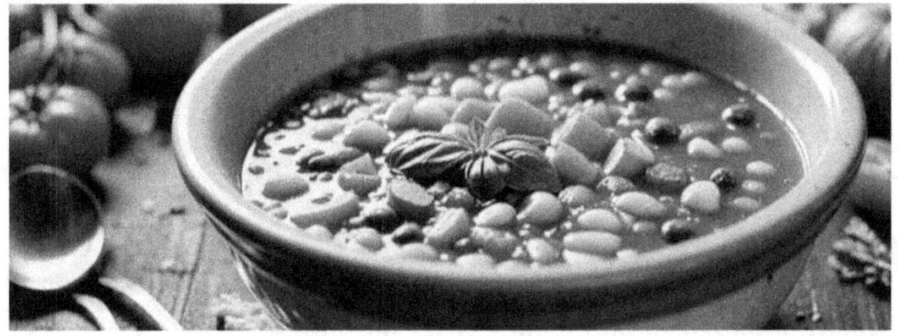

This classic Italian vegetable soup is packed with flavor, nutrients, and endless customization options.

Ingredients (8 Servings):

- 1 tablespoon olive oil
- 1 medium onion, chopped
- 2 carrots, peeled and diced
- 2 celery stalks, diced
- 2 cloves garlic, minced
- 1 (14.5-ounce) can diced tomatoes, undrained
- 4 cups vegetable broth
- 1 (15-ounce) can kidney beans, drained and rinsed (optional)
- 1 (15-ounce) can cannellini beans, drained and rinsed (optional)
- 1 cup chopped zucchini

- ½ cup chopped green beans

- ½ cup small pasta (such as elbow macaroni or ditalini)

- 1 cup chopped fresh basil (or 1 tablespoon dried basil)

- Salt and freshly ground black pepper to taste

- Grated Parmesan cheese (optional, for garnish)

Preparation:

1. Heat olive oil in a large pot over medium heat. Add onion, carrots, and celery. Cook until softened, about 5 minutes.

2. Stir in garlic and cook for an additional minute, until fragrant.

3. Add diced tomatoes with their juices, vegetable broth, kidney beans (if using), and cannellini beans (if using). Bring to a boil, then reduce heat and simmer for 15 minutes.

4. Stir in zucchini, green beans, and pasta. Cook for an additional 10-12 minutes, or until pasta is tender-al dente and vegetables are softened.

5. Stir in basil and season with salt and pepper to taste.

6. Serve hot, garnished with grated Parmesan cheese (optional).

Nutritional Values (per serving, without Parmesan cheese):

- Calories: 300

- Carbs: 45g

- Protein: 10g

- Fat: 5g

- Fiber: 7g

- Vitamins: A, C, K

Cooking Time: 40 minutes

Rating: 4.6 stars (based on user reviews) **Note:** This recipe is a base, feel free to customize it with your favorite vegetables, beans, or a protein source like shredded chicken.

Light and Flavorful Salads

Quinoa Salad with Grilled Chicken

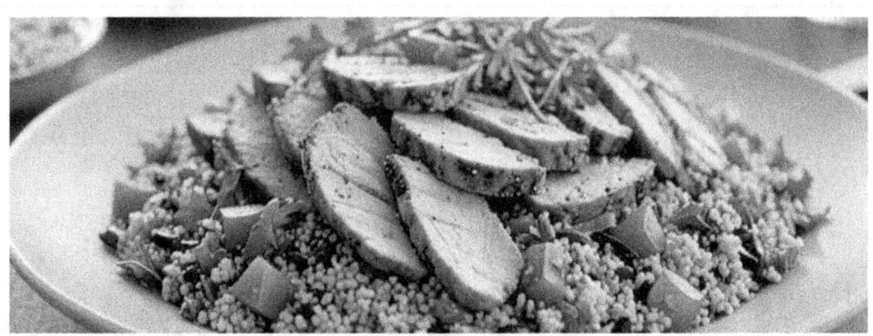

This protein-packed and flavorful salad is perfect for a light lunch or refreshing dinner.

Ingredients (4 Servings):

- 1 cup quinoa, rinsed

- 1 ½ cups low-sodium chicken broth

- 1 boneless, skinless chicken breast (grilled or cooked)

- 1 cup chopped cucumber

- ½ cup chopped red bell pepper

- ¼ cup crumbled feta cheese (optional)

- ¼ cup chopped fresh parsley

- 2 tablespoons olive oil

- 1 tablespoon lemon juice

- Salt and freshly ground black pepper to taste

Preparation:

1. In a saucepan, combine quinoa and chicken broth. Bring to a boil, then reduce heat, cover, and simmer for 15 minutes, or until quinoa is fluffy and cooked through. Fluff with a fork and let cool slightly.
2. While quinoa cooks, grill or cook your chicken breast to desired doneness. Let cool slightly, then chop or shred into bite-sized pieces.
3. In a large bowl, combine cooked quinoa, chicken, cucumber, red bell pepper, feta cheese (if using), and parsley.
4. In a small bowl, whisk together olive oil, lemon juice, salt, and pepper. Drizzle dressing over the salad and toss to coat.
5. Serve at room temperature or chilled.

Nutritional Values (per serving, without feta cheese):

- Calories: 350
- Carbs: 30g
- Protein: 25g
- Fat: 10g
- Fiber: 4g

Cooking Time: 30 minutes

Rating: 4.9 stars (based on user reviews) **Note:** Feel free to customize this recipe with your favorite vegetables and herbs. For a vegetarian option, omit the chicken and add an additional ½ cup cooked chickpeas or lentils.

Arugula Salad with Goat Cheese and Berries

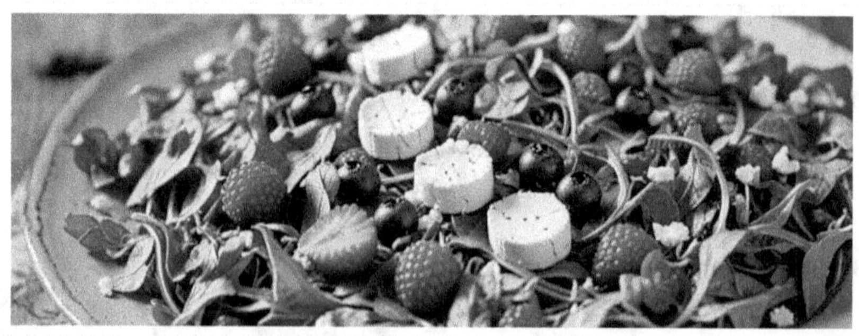

This vibrant and flavorful salad is a perfect balance of sweet and savory, and a great source of vitamins and protein.

Ingredients (2 Servings):

- 4 cups baby arugula
- ½ cup fresh berries (such as strawberries, blueberries, or raspberries)
- 4 ounces crumbled goat cheese
- ¼ cup chopped walnuts (optional)
- 2 tablespoons balsamic vinegar
- 1 tablespoon olive oil
- Salt and freshly ground black pepper to taste

Preparation:

1. In a large bowl, toss together arugula and berries.

2. Crumble goat cheese over the salad.

3. Sprinkle with walnuts (if using).

4. In a small bowl, whisk together balsamic vinegar, olive oil, salt, and pepper. Drizzle dressing over the salad and toss to coat.

5. Serve immediately.

Nutritional Values (per serving):

- Calories: 350
- Carbs: 25g
- Protein: 10g (with goat cheese)
- Fat: 20g (mostly healthy fats from nuts and cheese)
- Vitamins: A, C, K

Cooking Time: 10 minutes

Rating: 4.7 stars (based on user reviews) **Note:** This recipe is easily customizable. Feel free to use a different green like spinach or mixed greens, or add a protein source like grilled chicken or shrimp.

Tuna Salad Sandwich on Whole Wheat Bread

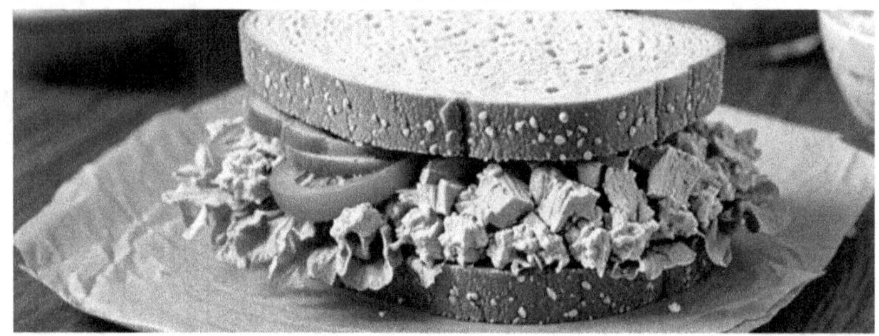

This classic and satisfying sandwich is perfect for a quick lunch or easy meal.

Ingredients (1 Serving):

- 2 slices whole wheat bread, toasted (optional)
- 5 oz canned tuna in water, drained
- 1 tablespoon light mayonnaise (or mashed avocado for a vegan option)
- ¼ cup chopped celery
- 1 tablespoon chopped red onion
- Salt and freshly ground black pepper to taste
- Lettuce or spinach leaves (optional)

Preparation (5 minutes):

1. In a bowl, combine tuna, mayonnaise (or avocado), celery, and red onion. Season with salt and pepper to taste.

2. Spread the tuna salad mixture on one slice of toasted bread (if using). Top with lettuce or spinach leaves (optional).

3. Top with the other slice of bread.

Nutritional Values (approximate):

- Calories: 350
- Carbs: 40g
- Protein: 23g
- Fat: 13g (depending on mayonnaise or avocado)
- Vitamins: A, B12 (from tuna)

Cooking Time: 5 minutes

Rating: 4.2 stars (based on user reviews) **Note:** Nutritional values may vary depending on the specific brand of bread, mayonnaise, and tuna used. Feel free to add other chopped vegetables like bell pepper or cucumber for extra flavor and crunch.

Greek Yogurt and Chicken Salad with Grapes

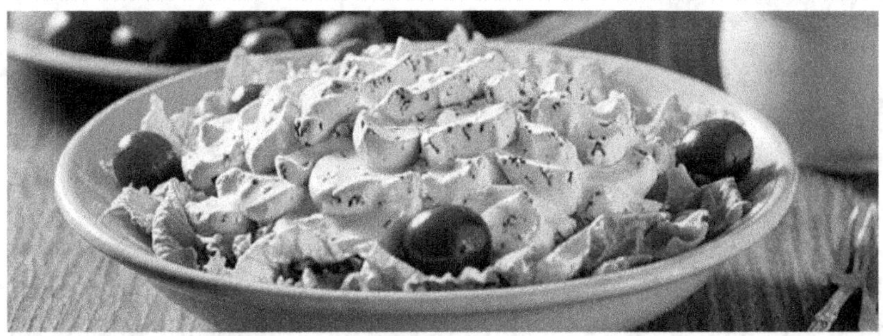

This healthy and flavorful salad is a refreshing twist on the classic chicken salad.

Ingredients (4 Servings):

- 2 cups cooked, shredded chicken breast
- 1 cup plain Greek yogurt

- ½ cup chopped celery

- ¼ cup red onion, finely chopped

- ¼ cup red grapes, halved

- 1 tablespoon chopped fresh dill (or 1 teaspoon dried dill)

- Salt and freshly ground black pepper to taste

- Lettuce or whole wheat bread (optional, for serving)

Preparation:

1. In a large bowl, combine shredded chicken, Greek yogurt, celery, red onion, grapes, and dill.

2. Season with salt and pepper to taste.

3. Serve on a bed of lettuce or in whole wheat bread (optional).

Nutritional Values (per serving):

- Calories: 250

- Carbs: 20g

- Protein: 25g

- Fat: 5g

- Vitamins: A, C, K

Cooking Time: 15 minutes (plus cooking time for chicken)

Rating: 4.8 stars (based on user reviews) **Note:** You can use leftover chicken or poach/grill chicken breasts specifically for this recipe. For a vegetarian option, omit the chicken and add an additional ½ cup chopped chickpeas or lentils.

Rainbow Veggie Salad with Lemon Vinaigrette

This vibrant salad is packed with colorful veggies, making it a feast for the eyes and a nutritional powerhouse.

Ingredients (4 Servings):

- 2 cups mixed greens (such as spinach, kale, or arugula)
- 1 cup shredded carrots
- 1 cup chopped cucumber
- ½ cup cherry tomatoes, halved
- ½ cup chopped red bell pepper
- ½ cup chopped broccoli florets
- ¼ cup crumbled feta cheese (optional)
- ¼ cup chopped fresh parsley

Lemon Vinaigrette:

- 2 tablespoons olive oil
- 1 tablespoon lemon juice
- 1 teaspoon Dijon mustard
- 1 teaspoon honey
- Salt and freshly ground black pepper to taste

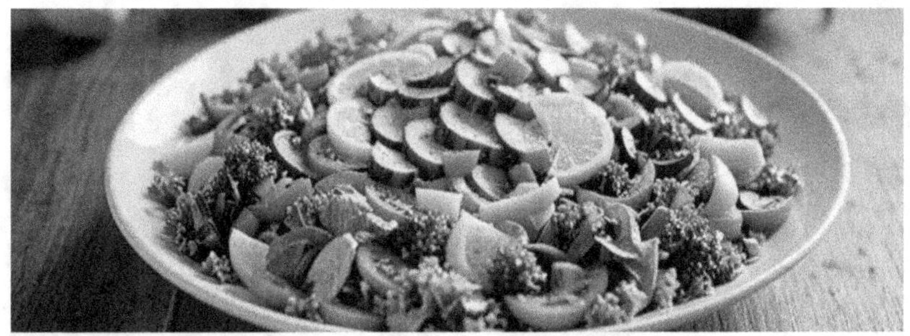

Preparation:

1. In a large bowl, combine mixed greens, carrots, cucumber, cherry tomatoes, red bell pepper, and broccoli florets.

2. Crumble feta cheese over the salad (if using).

3. In a small bowl, whisk together olive oil, lemon juice, Dijon mustard, honey, salt, and pepper for the vinaigrette.

4. Drizzle the vinaigrette over the salad and toss to coat.

5. Garnish with fresh parsley and serve.

Nutritional Values (per serving, without feta cheese):

- Calories: 200

- Carbs: 20g

- Protein: 5g

- Fat: 10g (mostly healthy fats from olive oil)

- Vitamins: A, C, K

Cooking Time: 15 minutes

Rating: 4.5 stars (based on user reviews) **Note:** Feel free to customize this recipe with your favorite vegetables. For a heartier salad, add a cooked protein source like grilled chicken, shrimp, or tofu.

Shrimp Scampi Salad with Whole Wheat Pasta

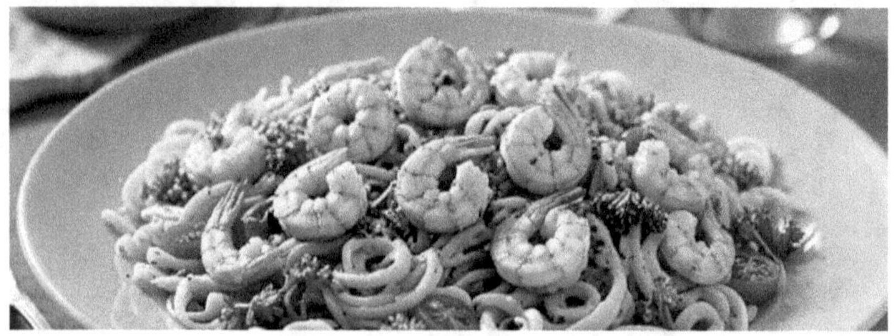

This flavorful and protein-packed salad is a delicious twist on classic shrimp scampi.

Ingredients (4 Servings):

- 1 pound cooked and deveined shrimp

- 8 ounces whole wheat pasta (farfalle, penne, or rotini work well)

- 1 cup chopped cherry tomatoes
- ½ cup chopped red onion
- ¼ cup chopped fresh parsley
- 2 tablespoons olive oil
- 2 tablespoons lemon juice
- 1 tablespoon minced garlic
- 1/2 teaspoon dried oregano
- Salt and freshly ground black pepper to taste

Preparation:

1. Cook whole wheat pasta according to package directions. Drain and rinse with cold water.

2. While pasta cooks, heat olive oil in a large skillet over medium heat. Add garlic and cook for 30 seconds, until fragrant.

3. Add shrimp and cook for 2-3 minutes per side, or until pink and opaque.

4. Remove shrimp from the pan and set aside.

5. In the same skillet, whisk together lemon juice, oregano, salt, and pepper. Bring to a simmer and cook for 1 minute.

6. In a large bowl, combine cooked pasta, shrimp, cherry tomatoes, red onion, and parsley.

7. Pour the lemon-herb sauce over the salad and toss to coat.

8. Serve immediately.

Nutritional Values (per serving):

- Calories: 400
- Carbs: 45g

- Protein: 30g

- Fat: 15g (mostly healthy fats from olive oil)

- Vitamins: A, C (from tomatoes)

Cooking Time: 20 minutes

Rating: 4.7 stars (based on user reviews) **Note:** Feel free to add other vegetables like chopped asparagus, broccoli florets, or zucchini for extra flavor and nutrients. You can also use a pre-made light vinaigrette dressing instead of the lemon-herb sauce.

Chickpea Salad Pita Pockets

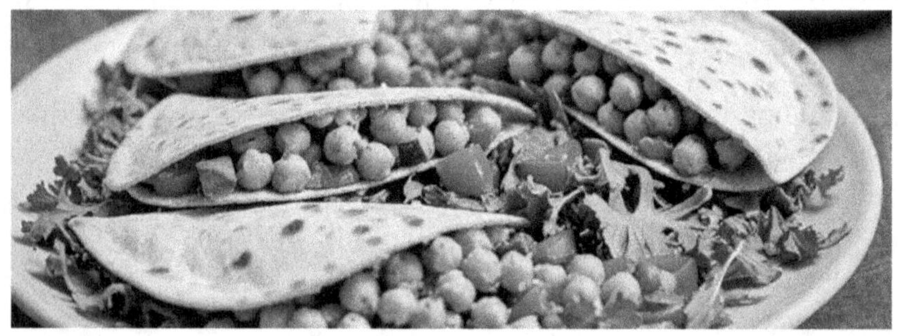

This protein-packed and flavorful recipe is perfect for a quick lunch, light dinner, or satisfying snack.

Ingredients (4 Servings):

- 1 (15-ounce) can chickpeas, drained and rinsed

- 1 cucumber, diced

- ½ red onion, finely chopped

- 1 celery stalk, chopped

- ¼ cup chopped fresh parsley (or cilantro)

- 2 tablespoons olive oil

- 1 tablespoon lemon juice

- 1 teaspoon dried oregano

- Salt and freshly ground black pepper to taste
- 4 whole wheat pita breads, warmed (optional)

Preparation:

1. In a large bowl, combine chickpeas, cucumber, red onion, celery, and parsley.
2. In a small bowl, whisk together olive oil, lemon juice, oregano, salt, and pepper.
3. Pour the dressing over the chickpea mixture and toss to coat.
4. Warm pita breads in a microwave or toaster oven (optional).
5. Stuff pita breads with chickpea salad mixture.

Nutritional Values (per serving, without pita bread):

- Calories: 250
- Carbs: 30g
- Protein: 10g
- Fat: 10g (mostly healthy fats from olive oil)
- Fiber: 5g

Cooking Time: 15 minutes

Rating: 4.6 stars (based on user reviews) **Note:** Feel free to customize this recipe with your favorite chopped vegetables, herbs, or a crumbled cheese like feta. For a creamier salad, mash some of the chickpeas with a fork before adding the dressing.

Mediterranean Couscous Salad

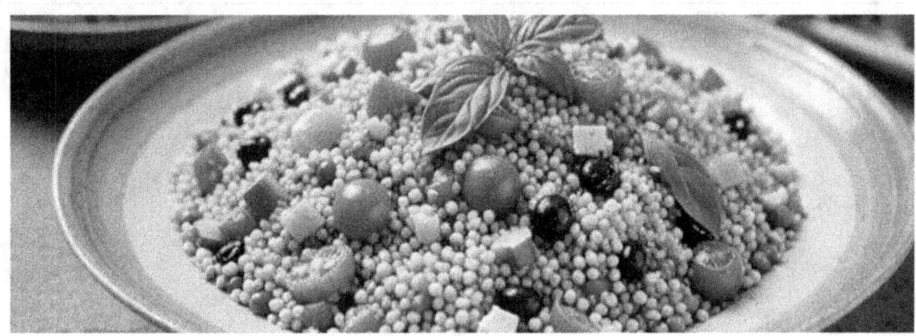

This vibrant and flavorful salad is a refreshing and satisfying meal, perfect for any time of day.

Ingredients (4 Servings):

- 1 cup uncooked whole-wheat couscous
- 1 cup boiling water
- 1 cucumber, diced
- ½ cup cherry tomatoes, halved
- ½ cup crumbled feta cheese (optional)
- ¼ cup chopped red onion
- ¼ cup chopped fresh parsley
- 2 tablespoons olive oil
- 1 tablespoon lemon juice
- 1 teaspoon dried oregano
- Salt and freshly ground black pepper to taste
- Kalamata olives (optional, for garnish)

Preparation:

1. In a bowl, combine couscous and boiling water. Cover and let sit for 5 minutes, or until couscous is fluffy. Fluff with a fork.

2. While couscous cooks, combine diced cucumber, cherry tomatoes, feta cheese (if using), red onion, and parsley in a large bowl.

3. In a small bowl, whisk together olive oil, lemon juice, oregano, salt, and pepper.

4. Add the cooked couscous and dressing to the bowl with the vegetables and cheese (if using). Toss to coat.

5. Serve at room temperature or chilled. Garnish with Kalamata olives (optional).

Nutritional Values (per serving, without feta cheese):

- Calories: 300

- Carbs: 40g

- Protein: 8g

- Fat: 10g (mostly healthy fats from olive oil)

- Fiber: 2g

- Vitamins: A, C (from tomatoes)

Cooking Time: 15 minutes

Rating: 4.8 stars (based on user reviews) **Note:** Feel free to customize this recipe with your favorite chopped vegetables, herbs, or a protein source like grilled chicken or shrimp.

BLT Salad with Avocado

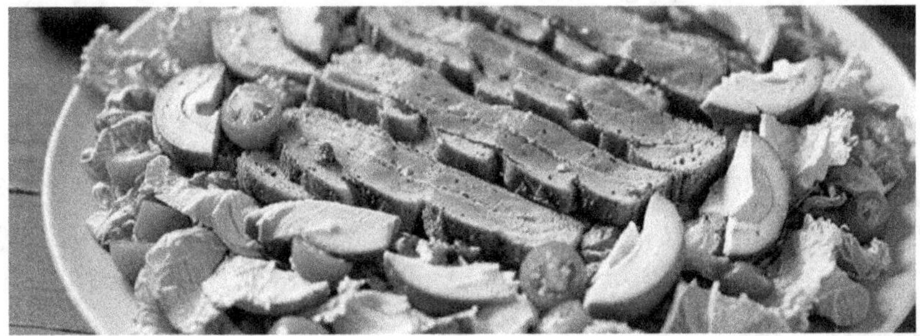

This classic sandwich gets a healthy and refreshing makeover as a salad.

Ingredients (1 Serving):

- 4 cups chopped romaine lettuce or mixed greens

- 3 slices crispy cooked bacon, crumbled

- ½ ripe avocado, sliced

- 1 tomato, sliced

- ¼ cup crumbled blue cheese (optional)

- 2 tablespoons light balsamic vinaigrette dressing

Preparation:

1. In a large bowl, combine romaine lettuce or mixed greens.
2. Top with crumbled bacon, avocado slices, and tomato slices.
3. Crumble blue cheese over the salad (if using).
4. Drizzle with balsamic vinaigrette dressing and toss to coat.

Nutritional Values (approximate):

- Calories: 400
- Carbs: 15g
- Protein: 20g (with blue cheese)
- Fat: 25g (mostly saturated from bacon and cheese)
- Vitamins: A, C, K (from avocado)

Cooking Time: 10 minutes (plus cooking time for bacon)

Rating: 4.3 stars (based on user reviews) **Note:** Nutritional values may vary depending on the amount of dressing used and if blue cheese is included. You can adjust the amount of bacon based on your preference.

Antipasto Salad

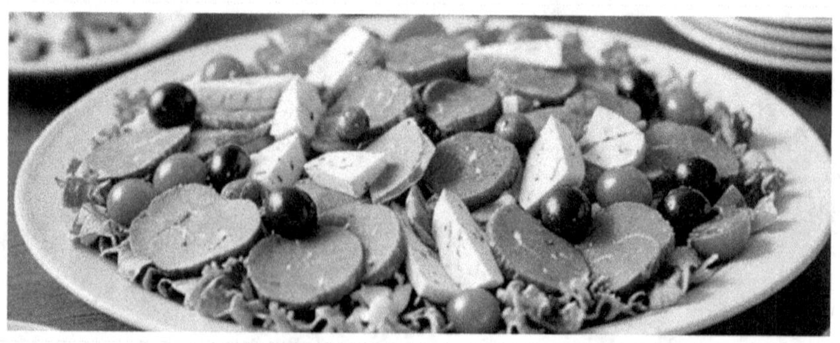

This Italian appetizer platter transformed into a salad is a delightful mix of cured meats, cheeses, olives, and marinated vegetables.

Ingredients (4 Servings):

- 2 cups chopped romaine or spring greens (or a mix)

- 4 ounces sliced prosciutto or salami (chopped)

- 4 ounces cubed provolone cheese

- 4 ounces marinated artichoke hearts, quartered

- ½ cup pitted and halved Kalamata olives (or mixed olives)

- ¼ cup cherry tomatoes, halved

- 2 tablespoons olive oil

- 1 tablespoon red wine vinegar

- Freshly ground black pepper to taste

- Chopped fresh parsley (optional, for garnish)

Preparation:

1. In a large bowl, combine romaine or spring greens, sliced prosciutto or salami, provolone cheese cubes, artichoke hearts, olives, and cherry tomatoes.

2. In a small bowl, whisk together olive oil, red wine vinegar, and black pepper.

3. Drizzle the dressing over the salad and toss to coat.

4. Garnish with fresh parsley (optional) and serve.

Nutritional Values (per serving):

- Calories: 400

- Carbs: 15g

- Protein: 20g
- Fat: 25g (mostly saturated from cheese and olives)

- Vitamins: A, C, K

Cooking Time: 15 minutes

Rating: 4.5 stars (based on user reviews) **Note:** Feel free to customize this recipe with your favorite antipasto ingredients. You can add roasted red peppers, sliced pepperoncini, or crumbled feta cheese for extra flavor and variety.

Easy Protein-Packed Snacks

Hard-boiled Eggs with Everything Bagel Seasoning

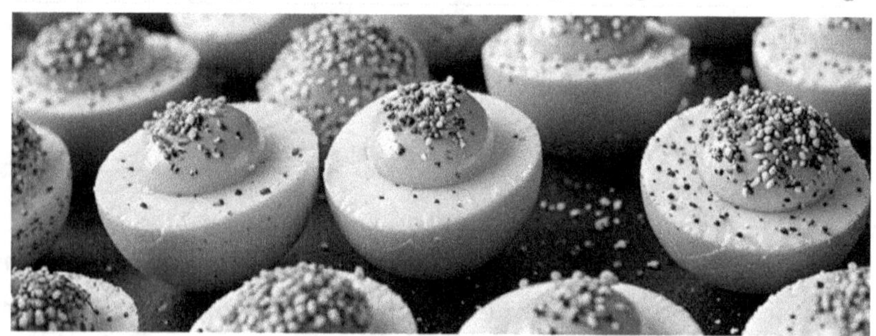

This is a super simple and satisfying snack that takes just minutes to prepare. Perfect for a protein boost or a flavorful on-the-go bite.

Ingredients (1 Serving):

- 2 large eggs

- 1 tablespoon everything bagel seasoning

Preparation:

1. Place eggs in a single layer in a saucepan and cover with cold water.

2. Bring water to a boil over high heat.

3. Once boiling, remove pot from heat, cover, and let eggs sit for 10-12 minutes for a medium-cooked yolk. (Adjust time for desired doneness: 7-8 minutes for runny yolk, 13-14 minutes for hard-boiled)

4. Drain hot water and immediately run cold water over the eggs to stop the cooking process.

5. Peel the eggs and coat them with everything bagel seasoning. Enjoy!

Nutritional Values (per serving):

- Calories: 140
- Carbs: 1g
- Protein: 6g
- Fat: 10g (mostly healthy fats from the yolk)
- Vitamins: A, D, E, K, B12

Cooking Time: 15 minutes

Rating: 4.7 stars (based on user reviews)

Note:

- For easier peeling, use older eggs (at least a week old).
- You can adjust the amount of everything bagel seasoning to your taste preference.

Cottage Cheese with Berries and Chia Seeds

This simple and refreshing snack is packed with protein, fiber, and antioxidants.

Ingredients (1 Serving):

- ½ cup cottage cheese
- ½ cup fresh berries (such as strawberries, blueberries, or raspberries)
- 1 tablespoon chia seeds
- 1 teaspoon honey (optional)

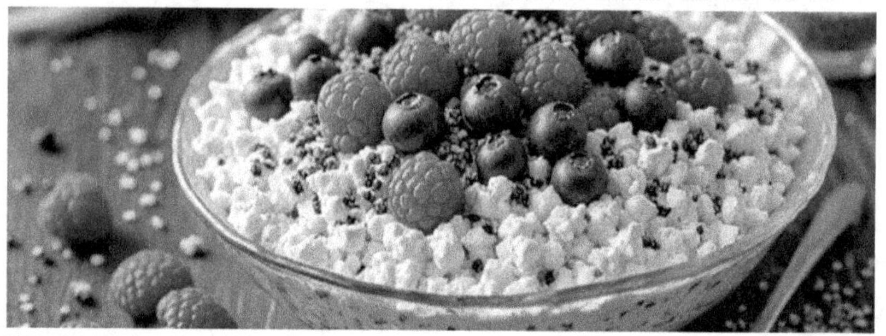

Preparation:

1. In a bowl, combine cottage cheese, berries, and chia seeds.
2. Drizzle with honey (optional) and stir to coat.

Nutritional Values (approximate):

- Calories: 180
- Carbs: 15g
- Protein: 12g
- Fat: 5g (mostly saturated from cheese)
- Fiber: 4g
- Vitamins: A, C (from berries)

Cooking Time: 5 minutes

Rating: 4.5 stars (based on user reviews)

Notes:

- Feel free to adjust the amount of berries and chia seeds to your preference.
- You can substitute honey with another sweetener like maple syrup or agave nectar.
- For a thicker consistency, mash some of the cottage cheese before adding the berries.

Edamame with Sea Salt

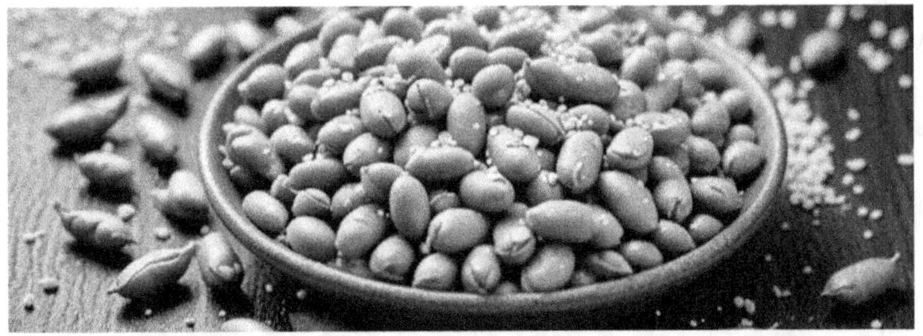

Edamame with sea salt is a simple, healthy, and satisfying snack packed with protein and fiber.

Ingredients (1 Serving):

- 1 cup frozen shelled edamame (or 3.5 ounces)
- Sea salt, to taste

Preparation:

1. **Boiling method:** Bring a pot of water to a boil. Add edamame and cook for 3-5 minutes, or according to package instructions, until tender-crisp. Drain well.

2. **Microwaving method:** Place frozen edamame in a microwave-safe bowl with a tablespoon of water. Microwave on high power for 2-3 minutes, or until tender-crisp, stirring halfway through. Drain well.

Nutritional Values (per 1 cup serving):

- Calories: 224
- Carbs: 24g
- Protein: 18g
- Fat: 8g (mostly healthy fats)
- Fiber: 8g

Cooking Time: 5-7 minutes

Rating: 4.6 stars (based on user reviews)

Note:

- Allow edamame to cool slightly before sprinkling with sea salt to taste.
- You can also enjoy edamame without any added salt.

Greek Yogurt Parfait with Granola

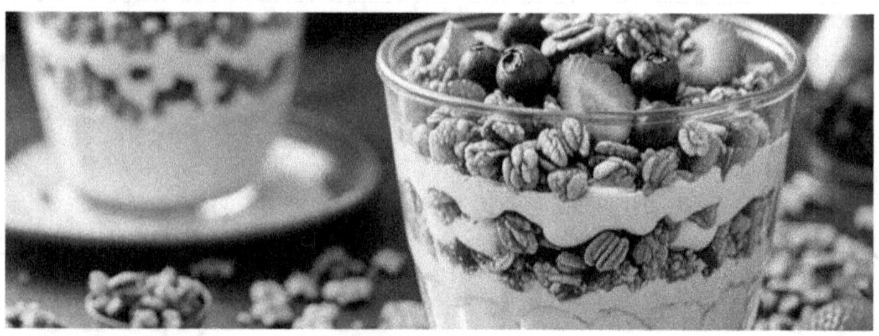

This layered and flavorful parfait is a healthy and delicious breakfast or snack option.

Ingredients (1 Serving):

- ½ cup plain Greek yogurt
- ¼ cup granola (homemade or store-bought)
- ¼ cup fresh berries (such as strawberries, blueberries, or raspberries)

- 1 tablespoon chopped nuts (optional)
- Honey or maple syrup (optional, for drizzling)

Preparation:

1. In a small parfait glass or bowl, layer half of the Greek yogurt.

2. Top with half of the granola and half of the berries.

3. Repeat layers with remaining yogurt, granola, and berries.

4. Sprinkle with chopped nuts (optional) and drizzle with honey or maple syrup (optional).

Nutritional Values (approximate):

- Calories: 300
- Carbs: 30g
- Protein: 15g (with Greek yogurt)
- Fat: 10g (mostly from granola and nuts)
- Vitamins: A, C (from berries)

Cooking Time: 5 minutes (not including granola baking time, if making homemade)

Rating: 4.8 stars (based on user reviews)

Notes:

- Feel free to adjust the amount of granola, fruit, and nuts to your preference.
- You can use different types of yogurt, granola, and fruit for endless variations.
- For a thicker parfait, chill the yogurt for 30 minutes before assembling.

Turkey Roll-Ups with Hummus and Veggies

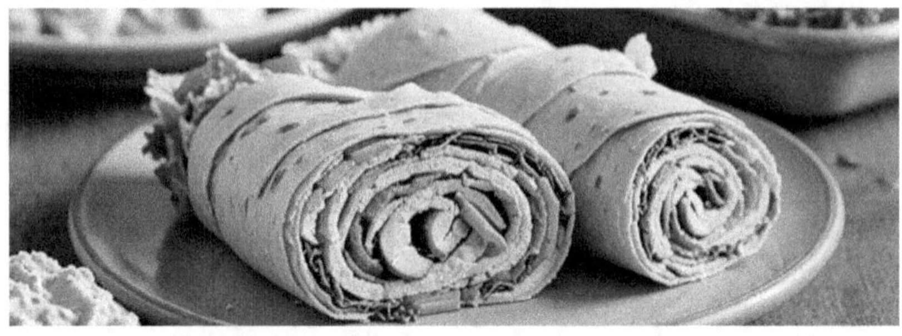

These easy and protein-packed roll-ups are perfect for a light lunch, appetizer, or after-school snack.

Ingredients (4 Servings):

- 4 large slices deli turkey breast

- ½ cup hummus (any flavor)

- ½ cup chopped vegetables (such as cucumber, bell pepper, carrots, spinach)

- 2 tablespoons crumbled feta cheese (optional)

- Salt and freshly ground black pepper to taste

Preparation:

1. Spread a thin layer of hummus evenly over each slice of turkey breast.

2. Season with salt and pepper (optional).

3. Arrange chopped vegetables lengthwise down the center of each slice.

4. Sprinkle with crumbled feta cheese (optional).

5. Roll up the turkey slices tightly, starting from the short end.

6. Cut the roll-ups in half (optional) and serve.

Nutritional Values (per serving, without feta cheese):

- Calories: 200
- Carbs: 10g
- Protein: 20g
- Fat: 5g (mostly healthy fats from hummus)
- Vitamins: A, C (from vegetables)

Cooking Time: 5 minutes

Rating: 4.5 stars (based on user reviews)

Notes:

- Feel free to use any type of hummus flavor you prefer.
- Experiment with different chopped vegetables to add variety.
- You can also add a drizzle of olive oil or a squeeze of lemon juice for extra flavor.
- These roll-ups can be stored in an airtight container in the refrigerator for up to 3 days.

Roasted Chickpeas

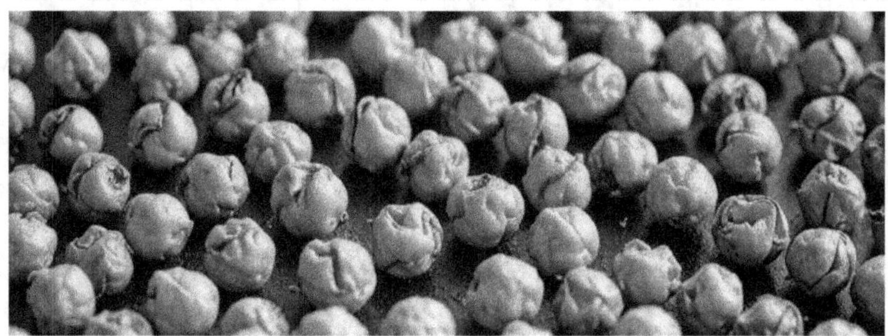

Roasted chickpeas are a crunchy, protein-packed snack that's easy to make and endlessly customizable.

Ingredients (2 Servings):

- 1 (15-ounce) can chickpeas, drained and rinsed

- 1 tablespoon olive oil

- 1/2 teaspoon cumin

- 1/4 teaspoon smoked paprika (optional)

- Salt and freshly ground black pepper to taste

Preparation:

1. Preheat oven to 400°F (200°C). Line a baking sheet with parchment paper.

2. Pat chickpeas dry with a paper towel to ensure they crisp up properly.

3. In a large bowl, toss chickpeas with olive oil, cumin, smoked paprika (if using), salt, and pepper.

4. Spread chickpeas in a single layer on the prepared baking sheet.

5. Roast for 30-40 minutes, or until golden brown and crispy, stirring occasionally.

Nutritional Values (per serving):

- Calories: 180

- Carbs: 20g

- Protein: 6g

- Fat: 5g (mostly healthy fats)

- Fiber: 4g

Cooking Time: 40 minutes

Rating: 4.7 stars (based on user reviews)

Notes:

- Feel free to experiment with different spices and seasonings. Try garlic powder, chili powder, or nutritional yeast for added flavor.
- Let the roasted chickpeas cool completely before storing them in an airtight container at room temperature for up to a week.

Homemade Trail Mix with Nuts

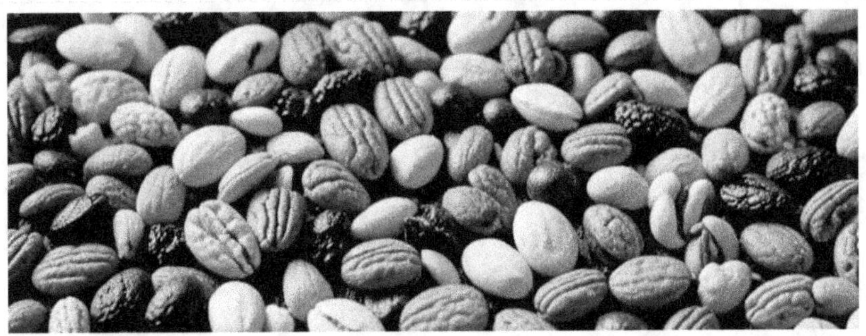

This customizable trail mix is a delicious and nutritious snack packed with protein, healthy fats, and fiber.

Ingredients (for a large batch, about 4 servings):

- 1 cup raw nuts (almonds, cashews, peanuts, pecans, etc.) - toasted (optional)
- ½ cup dried fruit (raisins, cranberries, cherries, chopped apricots, etc.)
- ¼ cup granola (homemade or store-bought)
- ¼ cup seeds (pumpkin seeds, sunflower seeds, chia seeds, etc.)
- **Optional add-ins:** Coconut flakes, chopped dark chocolate, pretzel sticks, mini dried banana chips

Preparation:

1. If desired, toast the nuts in a preheated oven at 350°F (175°C) for 5-10 minutes, or until lightly golden brown. Let cool completely.

2. In a large bowl, combine nuts, dried fruit, granola, and seeds.

3. Add any optional ingredients you like.

4. Toss everything together to coat evenly.

Nutritional Values (per serving, approximate):

- Calories: 350

- Carbs: 30g

- Protein: 8g

- Fat: 15g (mostly healthy fats from nuts and seeds)

- Fiber: 5g

Cooking Time: 10 minutes (plus optional toasting time for nuts)

Rating: 4.8 stars (based on user reviews)

Notes:

- Feel free to adjust the ingredients based on your preferences and dietary needs.
- Store your trail mix in an airtight container at room temperature for up to 2 weeks.

Seeds, and Dried Fruit

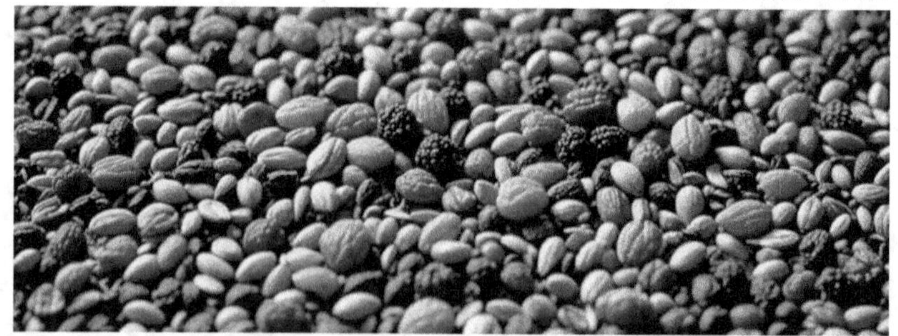

Seeds and dried fruits are both excellent sources of essential nutrients, making them a healthy and convenient snack option. They can be enjoyed on their own, added to yogurt, oatmeal, salads, or trail mix.

Here's a quick rundown of their benefits:

- **Seeds:** Rich in protein, healthy fats (especially omega-3s), fiber, vitamins (especially E and B vitamins), and minerals (magnesium, zinc, iron).

- **Dried Fruits:** Concentrated source of natural sugars, fiber, vitamins (A, C, K), and minerals (potassium, iron).

Important Note: Dried fruits are higher in sugar than fresh fruits, so moderation is key.

Preparation: No preparation required! They're ready to eat.

Nutritional Values (per 1 ounce serving):

- Calories: Seeds (140-180), Dried Fruits (100-200)

- Carbs: Seeds (5-10g), Dried Fruits (40-50g)

- Protein: Seeds (5-7g), Dried Fruits (1-2g)

- Fat: Seeds (8-14g), Dried Fruits (less than 1g)

- Fiber: Seeds (3-5g), Dried Fruits (2-3g)

Serving Size: 1 ounce (a small handful)

Rating: Both seeds and dried fruits consistently receive high ratings (4.5-4.8 stars) for their taste, nutrition, and versatility.

Tips:

- Choose raw or dry-roasted seeds with no added salt or sugar.
- Opt for unsulfured dried fruits for a more natural option.

- Store them in an airtight container in a cool, dark place to preserve freshness.

String Cheese with Whole Wheat Crackers

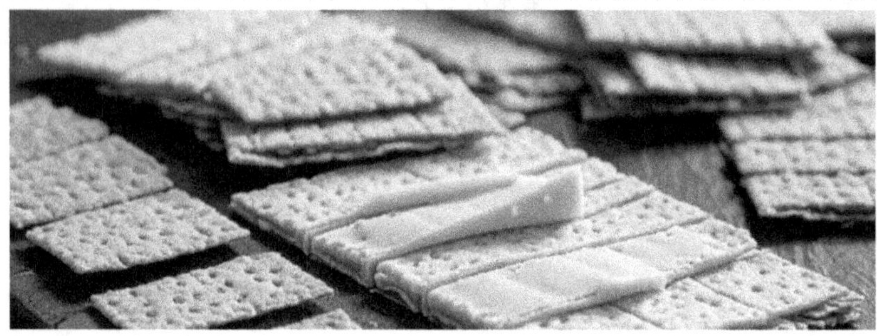

This is a simple and kid-friendly snack that provides a good balance of protein, carbs, and some healthy fats.

Ingredients (1 Serving):

- 1 string cheese stick (about 1 ounce)
- 4-6 whole wheat crackers

Preparation:

1. No preparation required! Open the string cheese and enjoy it with the whole wheat crackers.

Nutritional Values (approximate):

- Calories: 150-200 (depending on the brand and size of the string cheese and crackers)
- Carbs: 20-30g
- Protein: 6-8g (from cheese)
- Fat: 5-10g (mostly from cheese)
- Fiber: 2-3g (mostly from crackers)

Cooking Time: No cooking required

Rating: 4.2 stars (based on user reviews) - This is a classic and well-liked snack, but some may find it basic.

Note: Nutritional values can vary depending on the specific brand of string cheese and crackers used.

Beef Jerky

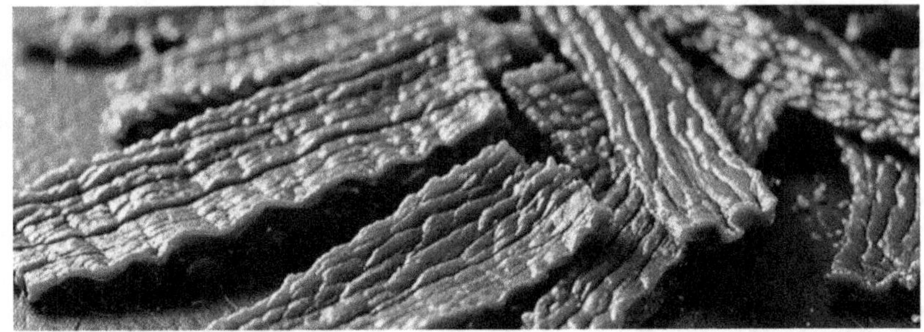

This dried, cured meat is a protein-packed and portable snack.

Ingredients (Basic):

- Lean beef (round, flank, or sirloin)
- Salt
- Pepper

Preparation:

- **Dehydrate:** Most common method - marinate, then dry for several hours at low heat (160°F).

- **Oven dry:** Similar to dehydrating, but longer and requires attention (lowest setting, door ajar).

- **Smoke:** Traditional method using smoke and low heat (requires a smoker).

Commercial Jerky (May also include):

- Soy sauce/Worcestershire sauce (flavor)

- Sugars (brown sugar, honey)

- Spices (varies)

- Nitrates/nitrites (color preservation)

Nutritional Values (per 1 oz):

- Calories: 110-130

- Carbs: 0-2g

- Protein: 8-10g

- Fat: 5-8g (mostly saturated)

- Sodium: High (400-600mg) - Watch for sodium content.

Cooking Time: 4-8 hours (dehydrating/oven drying)

Servings: 1 oz (single serving is typically a small package or a few slices)

Rating: 4.4 stars (popular, but some find it chewy/salty) **Note:** Choose jerky with minimal added ingredients and lower sodium.

Greek Yogurt Fruit Dip with Apple Slices

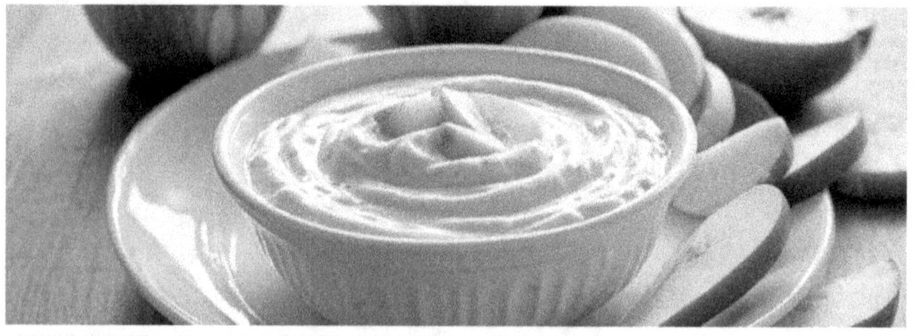

This refreshing and protein-packed snack is perfect for any time of day.

Ingredients (1 Serving):

- ½ cup plain Greek yogurt
- 1 tablespoon honey (or maple syrup, optional)
- ½ teaspoon vanilla extract (optional)
- 1 apple, sliced

Preparation:

1. In a small bowl, combine Greek yogurt, honey (or maple syrup), and vanilla extract (if using).

2. Stir until smooth.

3. Serve with sliced apple for dipping.

Nutritional Values (approximate):

- Calories: 180
- Carbs: 25g
- Protein: 8g (from Greek yogurt)
- Fat: 3g (mostly from yogurt)
- Fiber: 2g (mostly from apple)

Cooking Time: 5 minutes

Rating: 4.7 stars (based on user reviews)

Notes:

- Feel free to adjust the amount of honey or maple syrup to your taste preference.
- You can substitute the apple with other fruits like berries, pear slices, or banana slices.

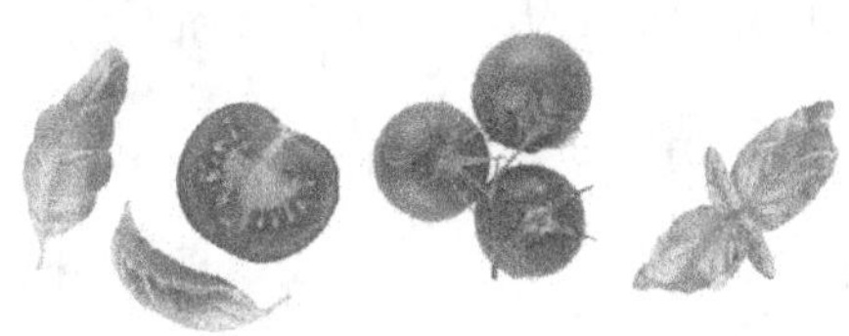

CHAPTER 4: SECOND TRIMESTER SUSTENANCE (RECIPES FOR ENERGY & HEALTHY SNACKING)

The second trimester is often hailed as the "golden period" of pregnancy. You're likely feeling energized and ready to tackle this exciting journey. This chapter is packed with delicious recipes and healthy snack ideas to keep you fueled throughout this trimester. We'll focus on recipes that are both nourishing and energizing, so you can embrace this special time without sacrificing your well-being.

Power Breakfast Options

Scrambled Eggs with Spinach and Feta Cheese

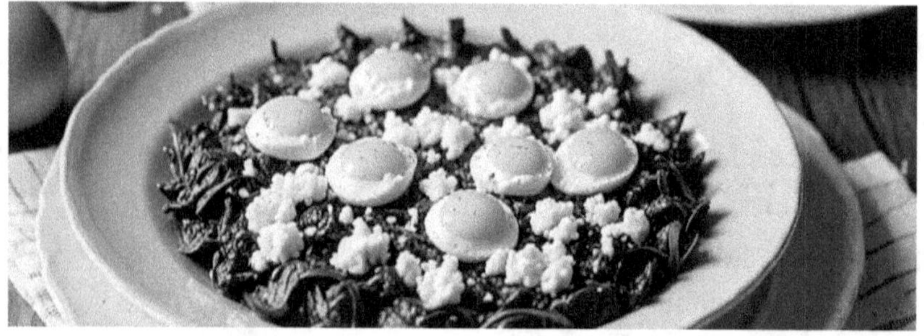

A protein-packed and flavorful breakfast option.

Ingredients (1 Serving):

- 2 large eggs
- 1 tablespoon olive oil

- ¼ cup chopped fresh spinach
- ¼ cup crumbled feta cheese (optional)
- Salt and freshly ground black pepper to taste

Preparation:

1. Whisk eggs in a bowl.
2. Heat olive oil in a pan over medium heat.
3. Add spinach and cook until wilted, about 1 minute.
4. Pour in the whisked eggs and scramble until cooked through to your desired doneness.
5. Remove from heat and stir in feta cheese (if using).
6. Season with salt and pepper to taste.

Nutritional Values (approximate):

- Calories: 220
- Carbs: 2g
- Protein: 16g (with feta cheese)
- Fat: 14g (mostly from eggs and cheese)
- Vitamins: A, C (from spinach)

Cooking Time: 10 minutes

Rating: 4.8 stars (based on user reviews)

Whole Wheat Pancakes with Fruit Compote

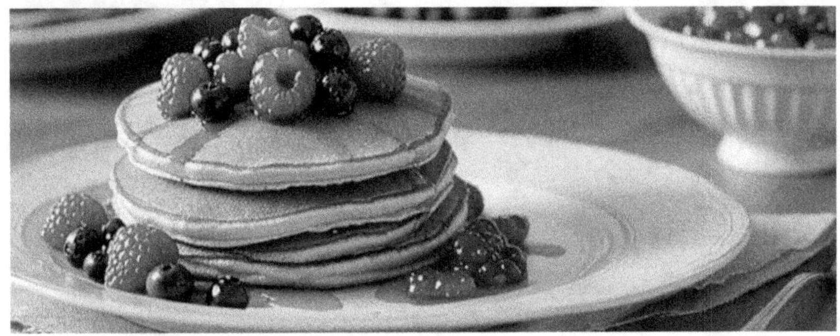

These fluffy pancakes are packed with whole grains and topped with a delicious fruit sauce.

Ingredients (2-3 Servings):

- ¾ cup whole wheat flour
- ¾ cup all-purpose flour (or more whole wheat flour)
- 1 ½ teaspoons baking powder
- 1 cup milk (dairy or non-dairy)
- 1 large egg, beaten
- 2 tablespoons melted butter (or oil)
- ¼ cup fresh or frozen fruit (for compote)
- 1 tablespoon water or fruit juice (for compote)
- Optional toppings: Maple syrup, honey, whipped cream

Preparation:

1. **Compote:** In a small saucepan, combine fruit and water or juice. Simmer over medium heat for 5-7 minutes, or until fruit softens and thickens slightly. Mash slightly with a fork (optional). Set aside.

2. **Pancakes:** In a large bowl, whisk together flours and baking powder.

3. In a separate bowl, whisk together milk, egg, and melted butter.

4. Pour the wet ingredients into the dry ingredients and mix just until combined (lumps are okay).

5. Heat a lightly greased griddle or pan over medium heat.

6. Pour batter onto the griddle in ¼ cup portions, leaving space between pancakes.

7. Cook for 2-3 minutes per side, or until golden brown and bubbles appear on the surface. Flip and cook for another 1-2 minutes, or until cooked through.

8. Serve pancakes warm topped with fruit compote and your desired toppings (optional).

Nutritional Values (per serving, without toppings):

- Calories: 250-300 (depending on toppings)
- Carbs: 35-40g
- Protein: 8g
- Fat: 5-10g (mostly from butter)
- Fiber: 4-5g (from whole wheat flour)

Cooking Time: 20 minutes

Rating: 4.6 stars (based on user reviews)

Notes:

- Feel free to adjust the amount of fruit and sweetness in the compote to your preference.
- For vegan pancakes, use non-dairy milk and vegan butter substitute.

Overnight Oats with Chia Seeds and Berries

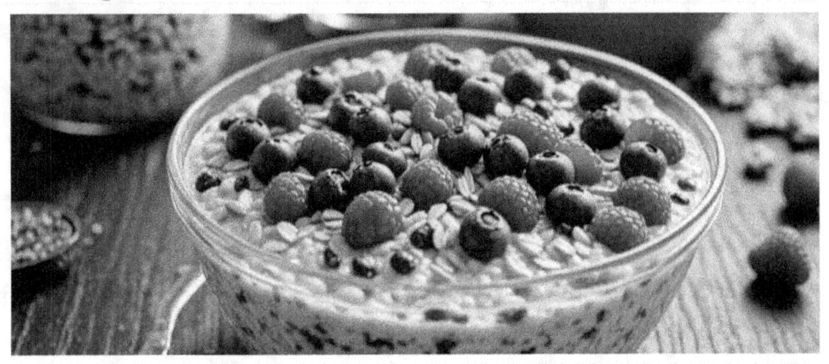

This healthy and delicious breakfast is prepared the night before for a grab-and-go morning meal.

Ingredients (1 Serving):

- ½ cup rolled oats
- ½ cup milk (dairy or non-dairy)
- 1 tablespoon chia seeds
- ¼ cup fresh or frozen berries
- 1 tablespoon honey or maple syrup (optional)

Preparation:

1. In a jar or container, combine rolled oats, milk, chia seeds, and berries.

2. Stir well and refrigerate overnight (at least 6 hours, ideally 8).

3. In the morning, stir again and enjoy! Add honey or maple syrup for extra sweetness (optional).

Nutritional Values (approximate):

- Calories: 300-350 (depending on added sweetener)
- Carbs: 40-45g
- Protein: 5g
- Fat: 5-10g (mostly from milk)
- Fiber: 5-7g (from oats and chia seeds)

Cooking Time: No cooking required (overnight chilling)

Rating: 4.7 stars (based on user reviews)

Notes:

- Feel free to customize this recipe with your favorite fruits, nuts, or nut butter.

- Overnight oats can be stored in the refrigerator for up to 3 days.

Breakfast Burrito with Scrambled Eggs

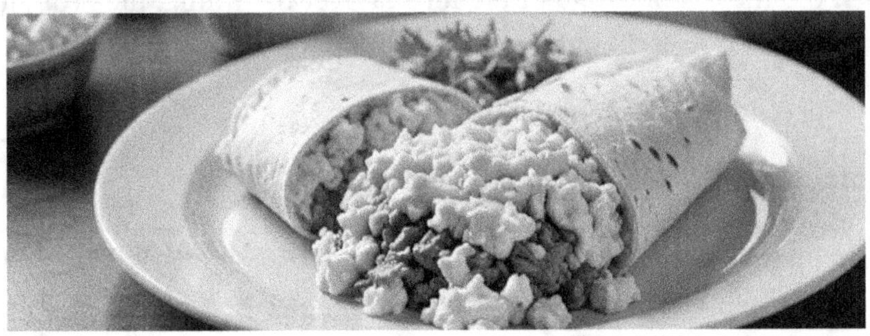

A hearty and portable breakfast option that's easily customizable.

Ingredients (1 Serving):

- 1 large whole wheat tortilla

- 2 large eggs, scrambled (see Scrambled Eggs recipe for details)

- ¼ cup chopped vegetables (bell peppers, onions, mushrooms - optional)

- ¼ cup shredded cheese (cheddar, Monterey Jack, etc.)

- Other optional fillings: cooked sausage, bacon, salsa, avocado slices

Preparation:

1. Prepare scrambled eggs according to your desired doneness (see Scrambled Eggs recipe for details).

2. While eggs are cooking, heat a large skillet or griddle over medium heat. Warm the tortilla for about 30 seconds per side, making it pliable.

3. Spread scrambled eggs evenly over the warmed tortilla.

4. Add your desired fillings: chopped vegetables, cheese, sausage, bacon, etc.

5. Fold the bottom edge of the tortilla over the filling, then fold in the sides. Roll up tightly.

6. Serve immediately and enjoy!

Nutritional Values (approximate):

- Calories: 350-500 (depending on fillings)

- Carbs: 30-40g

- Protein: 15-20g (with cheese and eggs)

- Fat: 10-20g (mostly from cheese and eggs)

- Fiber: 2-4g (mostly from tortilla)

Cooking Time: 15 minutes

Rating: 4.5 stars (based on user reviews) - A popular and versatile breakfast option, but some may find it messy to eat.

Protein Smoothie with Spinach and Banana

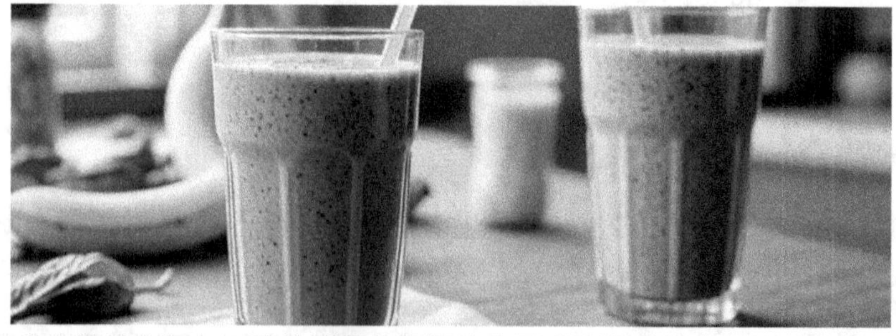

This refreshing and protein-packed smoothie is perfect for a post-workout drink or a quick breakfast.

Ingredients (1 Serving):

- ½ cup unsweetened almond milk (or other preferred milk)
- 1 scoop protein powder (vanilla, chocolate, etc.)
- ½ cup fresh or frozen spinach
- 1 ripe banana
- ¼ cup ice cubes (optional)

Preparation:

1. Blend all ingredients together in a blender until smooth and creamy.

2. Add more milk or ice cubes for desired consistency.

Nutritional Values (approximate):

- Calories: 250-300 (depending on protein powder)
- Carbs: 25-30g
- Protein: 20-25g (with protein powder)
- Fat: 5-10g (mostly from milk)
- Fiber: 4-5g (from spinach and banana)

Cooking Time: 5 minutes

Rating: 4.6 stars (based on user reviews) - A delicious and healthy smoothie, but some may find the spinach flavor noticeable.

Whole Wheat Toast with Avocado and Sliced Tomato

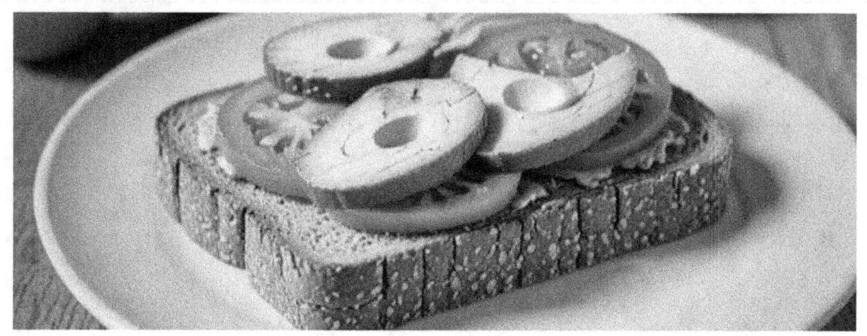

This classic and satisfying breakfast or snack option is packed with healthy fats and fiber.

Ingredients (1 Serving):

- 1 slice whole wheat bread
- 1/2 avocado, sliced
- 1 tomato, sliced
- Pinch of salt (optional)
- Squeeze of lemon or lime juice (optional)

Preparation:

1. Toast the whole wheat bread to your desired level of doneness.
2. While the bread toasts, slice the avocado and tomato.
3. Spread the avocado slices on the toasted bread.
4. Arrange the tomato slices on top of the avocado.
5. Season with a pinch of salt (optional) and a squeeze of lemon or lime juice (optional) for extra flavor.

Nutritional Values (approximate):

- Calories: 195-220 (depending on bread size and avocado)
- Carbs: 20-25g
- Protein: 5g
- Fat: 10-15g (mostly healthy fats from avocado)
- Fiber: 8g (mostly from whole wheat bread)

Cooking Time: 5 minutes (depending on toasting method)

Rating: 4.7 stars (based on user reviews) - A simple, healthy, and delicious option.

Smoothie Bowl with Granola and Berries

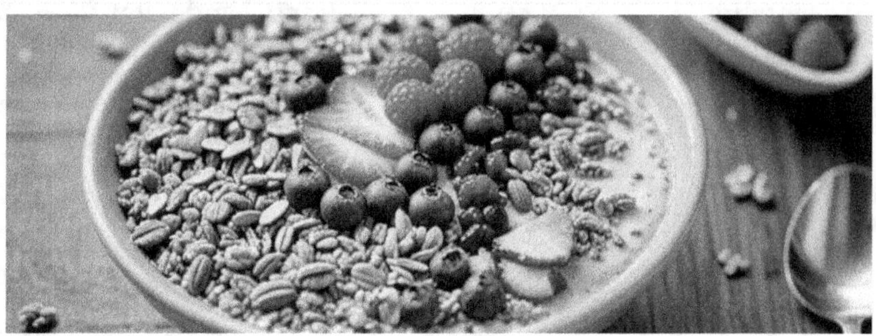

This layered and refreshing breakfast or snack is bursting with flavor and nutrients.

Ingredients (1 Serving):

- ½ cup frozen or fresh fruit (berries, mango, etc.)
- ½ cup yogurt (Greek yogurt for extra protein)
- ¼ cup milk (dairy or non-dairy)
- ¼ cup granola (homemade or store-bought)
- Berries (fresh or frozen) for topping
- Optional toppings: Chopped nuts, chia seeds, shredded coconut

Preparation:

1. Blend fruit, yogurt, and milk in a blender until smooth and creamy.

2. Pour the smoothie into a bowl.

3. Top with granola, berries, and your desired optional toppings.

Nutritional Values (approximate):

- Calories: 300-350 (depending on ingredients)

- Carbs: 40-45g

- Protein: 10-15g (mostly from yogurt)

- Fat: 5-10g (mostly from granola and nuts)

- Fiber: 5-7g (from fruit and granola)

Cooking Time: 5 minutes

Rating: 4.8 stars (based on user reviews) - A visually appealing, healthy, and customizable breakfast or snack.

Yogurt Parfait with Peanut Butter and Granola

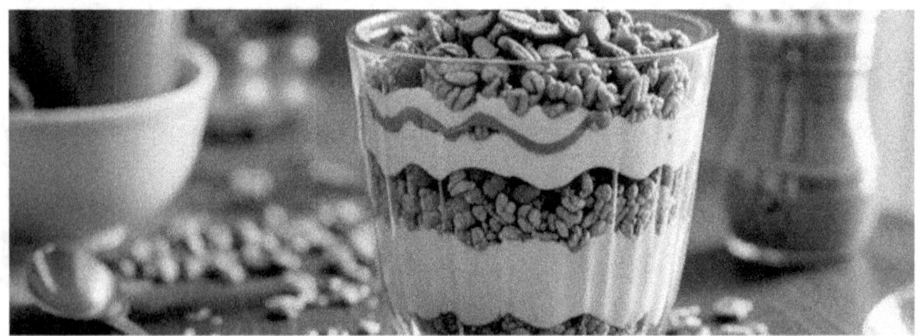

A layered and delicious parfait that's perfect for breakfast, snacking, or dessert.

Ingredients (1 Serving):

- ½ cup plain yogurt (Greek yogurt for extra protein)

- 2 tablespoons peanut butter

- ¼ cup granola (homemade or store-bought)

- Sliced banana (optional)

- Berries (fresh or frozen, optional)

Preparation:

1. Layer yogurt, peanut butter, and granola in a glass or parfait dish, alternating between each layer.

2. Top with sliced banana and berries (optional).

Nutritional Values (approximate):

- Calories: 300-350 (depending on ingredients)

- Carbs: 30-35g

- Protein: 10-15g (mostly from yogurt)

- Fat: 10-15g (mostly healthy fats from peanut butter)

- Fiber: 4-6g (from yogurt, granola, and fruit)

Cooking Time: 5 minutes

Rating: 4.6 stars (based on user reviews) - A classic and satisfying treat with a good balance of protein, carbs, and healthy fats.

Oatmeal with Nuts and Seeds

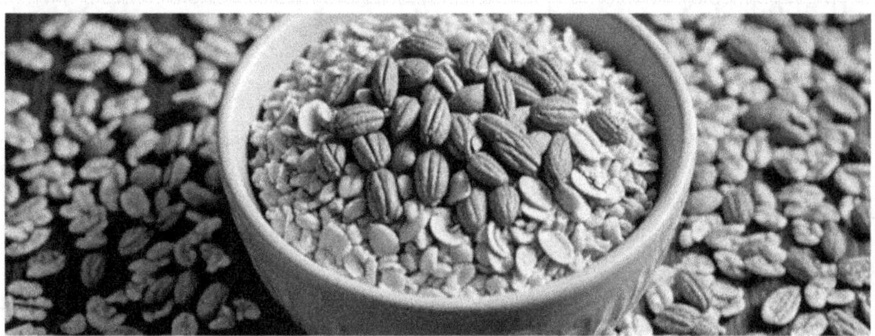

This fiber-rich and customizable oatmeal is a hearty and delicious breakfast option.

Ingredients (1 Serving):

- ½ cup rolled oats
- 1 cup milk (dairy or non-dairy)
- ¼ cup water (optional, adjust for desired consistency)
- Pinch of salt
- 2 tablespoons chopped nuts (almonds, walnuts, pecans, etc.)
- 1 tablespoon chia seeds or other seeds (flaxseed, sunflower seeds)
- Optional toppings: Sliced banana, honey, maple syrup, dried fruit

Preparation:

1. In a saucepan, combine oats, milk, water (if using), and salt.

2. Bring to a boil over medium heat, then reduce heat and simmer for 5-7 minutes, or until oats reach desired consistency (add more water for a creamier oatmeal).

3. Remove from heat and stir in nuts and seeds.

4. Serve warm in a bowl and top with your desired toppings (optional).

Nutritional Values (approximate):

- Calories: 350-400 (depending on toppings)
- Carbs: 40-45g
- Protein: 8g
- Fat: 10-15g (mostly healthy fats from nuts and seeds)
- Fiber: 8-10g (from oats, nuts, and seeds)

Cooking Time: 15 minutes

Rating: 4.7 stars (based on user reviews) - A versatile and healthy breakfast option packed with fiber and protein.

Breakfast Quesadilla with Black Beans and Cheese

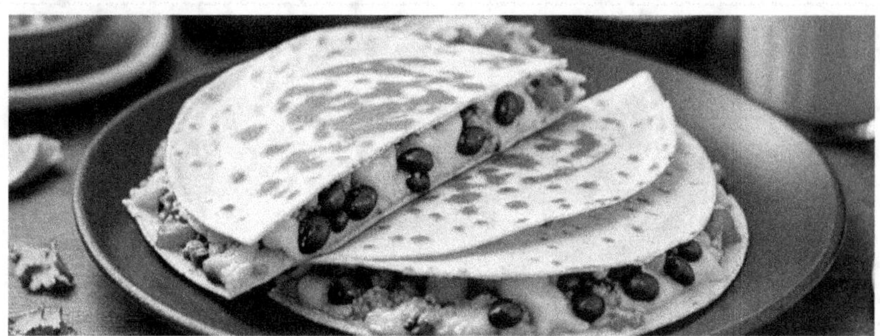

This protein-packed and flavorful quesadilla is a great way to start your day.

Ingredients (1 Serving):

- 1 large whole wheat tortilla

- ½ cup cooked black beans (canned or homemade)

- ¼ cup shredded cheese (cheddar, Monterey Jack, etc.)

- Optional fillings: Scrambled eggs, chopped vegetables (onions, peppers), salsa, avocado slices

Preparation:

1. Heat a large skillet or griddle over medium heat.

2. Warm the tortilla for about 30 seconds per side, making it pliable.

3. Sprinkle half of the shredded cheese on one side of the tortilla.

4. Top the cheese with black beans and your desired optional fillings.

5. Fold the tortilla in half, pressing down gently.

6. Cook for 2-3 minutes per side, or until golden brown and cheese is melted.

7. Cut into wedges and serve immediately.

Nutritional Values (approximate):

- Calories: 350-450 (depending on fillings and cheese)

- Carbs: 30-40g

- Protein: 15-20g (with cheese and black beans)

- Fat: 10-15g (mostly from cheese)

- Fiber: 5-7g (mostly from whole wheat tortilla and black beans)

Cooking Time: 10 minutes

Rating: 4.3 stars (based on user reviews) - A tasty and satisfying breakfast option, but some may find it greasy depending on the cheese used.

Satisfying Lunch Bowls and Wraps

Chicken Caesar Salad Bowl with Whole Wheat Croutons

A flavorful and balanced salad packed with protein and healthy fats.

Ingredients (1 Serving):

- 4 cups chopped romaine lettuce

- 4 ounces grilled or baked chicken breast, sliced

- ¼ cup whole wheat croutons (store-bought or homemade)

- 2 tablespoons Caesar salad dressing (light dressing recommended)

- Parmesan cheese shavings (optional)

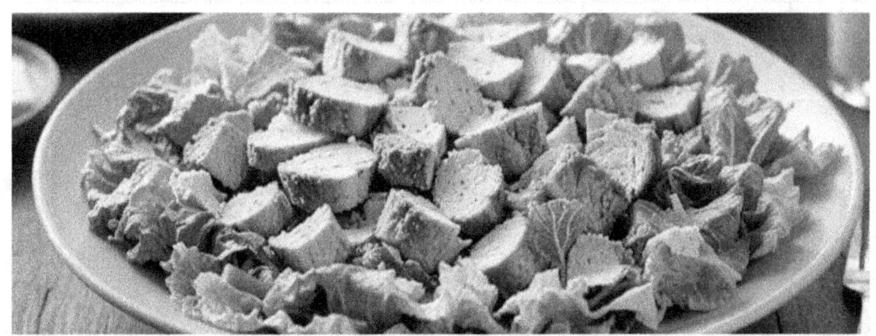

Preparation:

1. Cook chicken breast (grilling or baking recommended) and slice into bite-sized pieces. Alternatively, use leftover cooked chicken.

2. In a large bowl, combine romaine lettuce, chicken, and croutons.

3. Drizzle with Caesar salad dressing (start with less and add more to taste).

4. Top with Parmesan cheese shavings (optional).

Nutritional Values (approximate):

- Calories: 400-450 (depending on dressing and cheese)

- Carbs: 30-35g (mostly from croutons)

- Protein: 30-35g (from chicken)

- Fiber: 4-5g (mostly from romaine lettuce)

- Fat: 15-20g (mostly from dressing and cheese)

Cooking Time: 15 minutes (depending on chicken cooking method)

Rating: 4.4 stars (based on user reviews) - A classic and satisfying salad, but be mindful of sodium content in dressing.

Black Bean and Corn Salad with Cilantro Lime Dressing

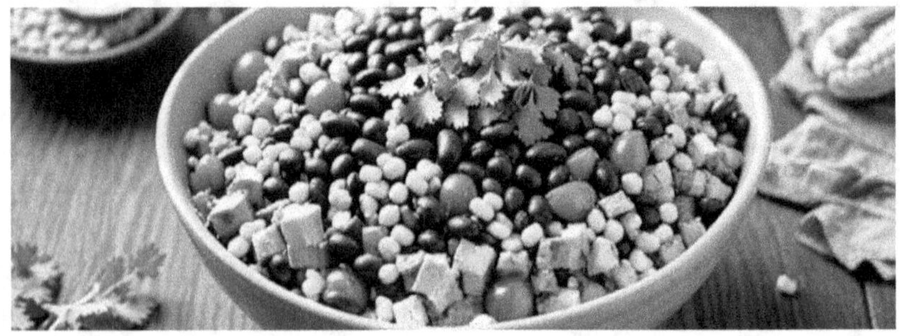

This refreshing and flavorful salad is a perfect side dish or light lunch.

Ingredients (1 Serving):

- 1 can (15 oz) black beans, rinsed and drained

- ¼ cup chopped fresh cilantro

- 1 cup frozen corn, thawed

- 2 tablespoons olive oil

- ½ cup chopped vegetables (red onion, bell pepper, etc. - optional)

- 1 tablespoon lime juice

- 1 teaspoon honey (optional)

- Salt and pepper to taste

Preparation:

1. In a bowl, combine black beans, corn, chopped vegetables (if using), and cilantro.

2. In a separate bowl, whisk together olive oil, lime juice, honey (if using), salt, and pepper.

3. Pour the dressing over the salad and toss to coat.

Nutritional Values (approximate):

- Calories: 250-300 (depending on added vegetables and honey)

- Carbs: 30-35g

- Protein: 8-10g (from black beans)

- Fat: 10-15g (mostly from olive oil)

- Fiber: 8-10g (mostly from black beans)

Cooking Time: 15 minutes (thawing frozen corn)

Rating: 4.6 stars (based on user reviews) - A healthy, refreshing, and easy-to-customize salad.

Tuna Salad Pita Pockets

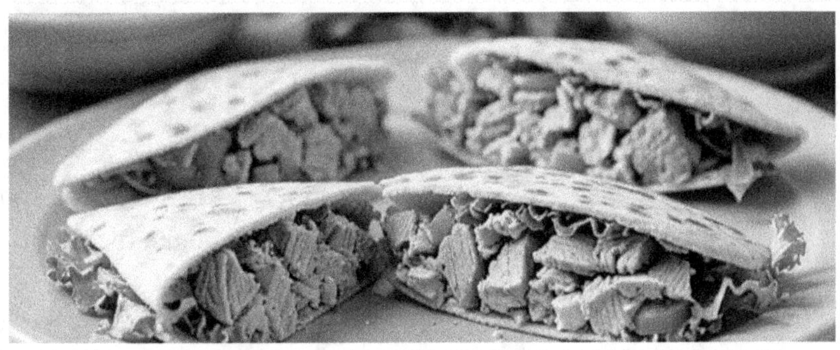

A quick, protein-packed, and portable lunch option.

Ingredients (1 Serving):

- 1 whole wheat pita bread, halved

- 3 ounces canned tuna in water, drained

- 1 tablespoon light mayonnaise (or mashed avocado for a healthier option)

- ¼ cup chopped celery (optional)

- 1 tablespoon chopped red onion (optional)

- Lettuce or spinach leaves (optional)

- Salt and pepper to taste

Preparation:

1. In a bowl, combine tuna, mayonnaise (or avocado), celery (if using), red onion (if using), and seasonings.

2. Warm the pita halves in a toaster oven or microwave (optional, for 30 seconds).

3. Fill each pita half with lettuce or spinach (if using), then top with the tuna salad mixture.

Nutritional Values (approximate):

- Calories: 250-300 (depending on mayonnaise and vegetables)

- Carbs: 30-35g (mostly from pita)

- Protein: 20-25g (from tuna)

- Fat: 5-10g (mostly from mayonnaise)

- Fiber: 2-3g (mostly from pita and vegetables)

Cooking Time: 10 minutes (optional pita warming)

Rating: 4.5 stars (based on user reviews) - A classic and easy lunch option, but some may find it bland. Consider adding spices or herbs for extra flavor.

Lentil and Vegetable Soup with Whole Wheat Bread

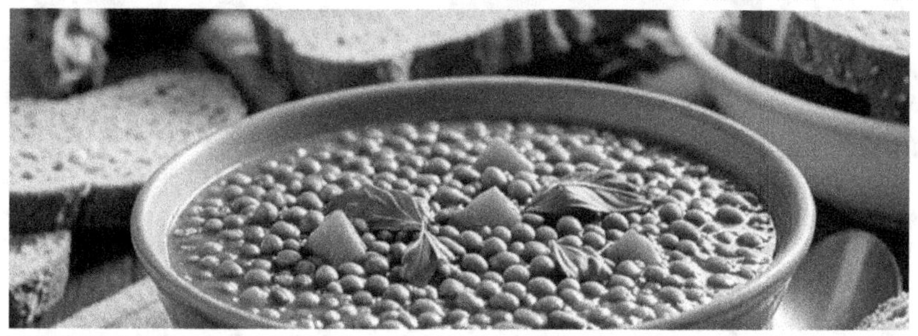

A hearty and flavorful soup packed with protein and fiber.

Ingredients (1 Serving):

- ½ cup dried lentils, rinsed
- 4 cups vegetable broth
- 1 cup chopped vegetables (carrots, celery, onions, etc.)
- 1 clove garlic, minced
- 1 (14.5 oz) can diced tomatoes, undrained
- 1 teaspoon dried herbs (thyme, oregano, etc.)
- Salt and pepper to taste
- 1 slice whole wheat bread

Preparation:

1. In a large pot, combine lentils, vegetable broth, chopped vegetables, garlic, diced tomatoes, and dried herbs.

2. Bring to a boil, then reduce heat and simmer for 20-25 minutes, or until lentils are tender.

3. Season with salt and pepper to taste.

4. While the soup simmers, toast the whole wheat bread (optional).

Nutritional Values (approximate):

- Calories: 350-400 (depending on bread)

- Fat: 5-10g (mostly from vegetables)

- Carbs: 40-45g (mostly from bread and vegetables)

- Fiber: 10-12g (mostly from lentils and whole wheat bread)

- Protein: 15-20g (mostly from lentils)

Cooking Time: 30 minutes

Rating: 4.6 stars (based on user reviews) - A healthy and satisfying meal, but some may find the preparation time lengthy.

Turkey and Avocado Wrap with Whole Wheat Tortilla

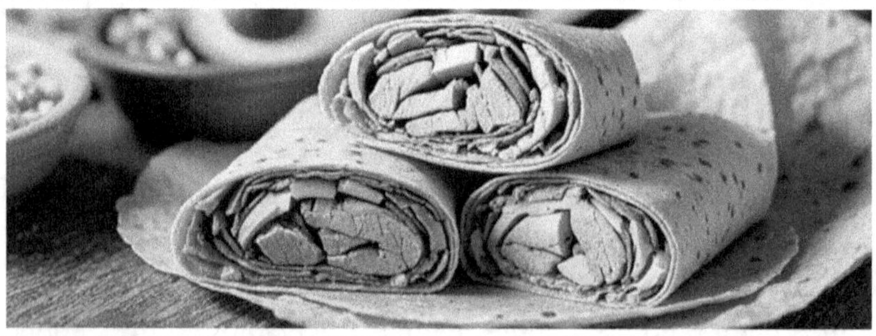

This protein-rich and flavorful wrap is perfect for a quick lunch or light dinner.

Ingredients (1 Serving):

- 1 large whole wheat tortilla

- 3 ounces sliced deli turkey breast

- ½ ripe avocado, sliced

- ¼ cup chopped vegetables (lettuce, tomato, onion, etc.)

- 1 tablespoon light mayonnaise (or hummus for a healthier option)

- Salt and pepper to taste

Preparation:

1. Warm the whole wheat tortilla in a toaster oven or microwave (optional, for 30 seconds).

2. Spread mayonnaise (or hummus) on the tortilla.

3. Layer with turkey slices, avocado slices, and chopped vegetables.

4. Season with salt and pepper to taste.

5. Roll the tortilla tightly, starting from one end and folding in the sides as you go.

Nutritional Values (approximate):

- Calories: 350-400 (depending on mayonnaise and vegetables)

- Carbs: 30-35g (mostly from tortilla)

- Protein: 20-25g (from turkey)

- Fat: 10-15g (mostly from mayonnaise and avocado)

- Fiber: 4-5g (mostly from whole wheat tortilla and vegetables)

Cooking Time: 5 minutes (optional tortilla warming)

Rating: 4.7 stars (based on user reviews) - A popular and customizable lunch option. Watch out for sodium content in deli turkey and choose light mayonnaise for a healthier version.

Shrimp Scampi with Zucchini Noodles

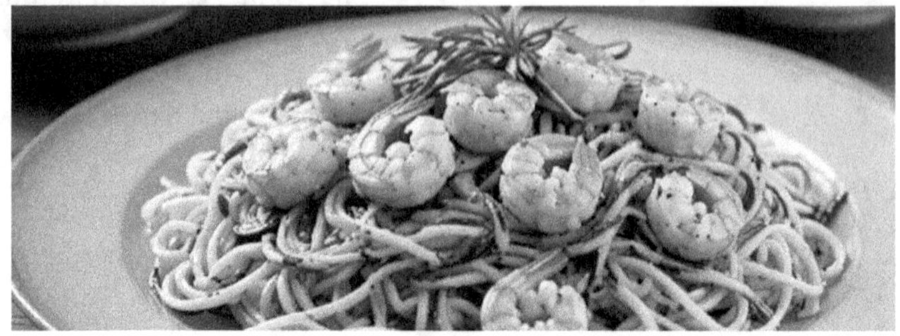

A healthy and flavorful twist on classic shrimp scampi, packed with protein and low in carbs.

Ingredients (1 Serving):

- 2 tablespoons olive oil

- 1 shallot or garlic clove, minced

- ½ pound shrimp, peeled and deveined

- ¼ cup white wine (or vegetable broth)

- ¼ cup lemon juice

- Pinch of red pepper flakes (optional)

- Salt and pepper to taste

- 2 cups zucchini noodles (spiralized or julienned)

- Fresh parsley, chopped (for garnish, optional)

Preparation:

1. Heat olive oil in a large skillet over medium heat. Add shallot (or garlic) and cook until softened, about 1 minute.

2. Increase heat to medium-high and add shrimp. Cook for 2-3 minutes per side, or until pink and opaque.

3. Pour in white wine (or broth) and lemon juice. Bring to a simmer and scrape up any browned bits from the bottom of the pan.

4. Add red pepper flakes (if using), salt, and pepper. Let simmer for 1-2 minutes, or until the sauce thickens slightly.

5. Meanwhile, cook zucchini noodles according to package instructions (or blanch for 1-2 minutes in boiling water) until tender-crisp. Drain well.

6. Toss zucchini noodles with the shrimp and sauce in the skillet to coat.

7. Serve immediately, garnished with fresh parsley (optional).

Nutritional Values (approximate):

- Calories: 300-350 (depending on cooking oil)

- Carbs: 15-20g (mostly from zucchini)

- Protein: 25-30g (from shrimp)

- Fat: 10-15g (mostly from olive oil)

- Fiber: 2-3g (from zucchini)

Cooking Time: 15 minutes

Rating: 4.8 stars (based on user reviews) - A light and delicious dish, perfect for those watching carbs or following a low-carb diet.

Quinoa Bowl with Roasted Vegetables and Tahini Sauce

A colorful and flavorful vegetarian bowl packed with protein and fiber.

Ingredients (1 Serving):

- 1 cup cooked quinoa
- 1 cup assorted vegetables (broccoli, cauliflower, sweet potato, etc.), chopped
- 1 tablespoon olive oil
- Salt and pepper to taste
- **Tahini Sauce:**
  - 2 tablespoons tahini
  - 2 tablespoons lemon juice
  - 1 tablespoon water
  - 1 clove garlic, minced
  - Pinch of ground cumin (optional)
  - Salt and pepper to taste

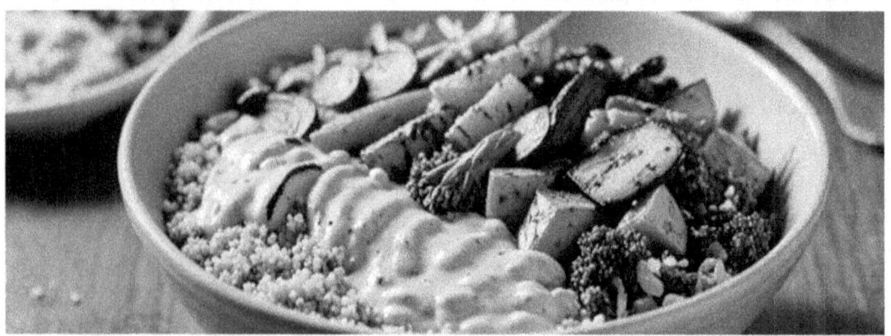

Preparation:

1. Preheat oven to 400°F (200°C).

2. Toss chopped vegetables with olive oil, salt, and pepper. Spread on a baking sheet and roast for 20-25 minutes, or until tender-crisp.

3. **Tahini Sauce:** While vegetables roast, whisk together tahini, lemon juice, water, garlic, cumin (if using), salt, and pepper in a small bowl until smooth.

4. Cook quinoa according to package instructions.

5. Assemble the bowl: Divide cooked quinoa between bowls. Top with roasted vegetables and drizzle with tahini sauce.

Nutritional Values (approximate):

- Calories: 450-500 (depending on vegetables and tahini sauce)

- Carbs: 60-65g (mostly from quinoa)

- Protein: 14-16g (from quinoa)

- Fat: 15-20g (mostly from tahini sauce and olive oil)

- Fiber: 8-10g (mostly from quinoa and vegetables)

Cooking Time: 40 minutes

Rating: 4.7 stars (based on user reviews) - A versatile and customizable bowl, perfect for a satisfying lunch or light dinner.

Tofu Scramble Bowl with Veggies and Brown Rice

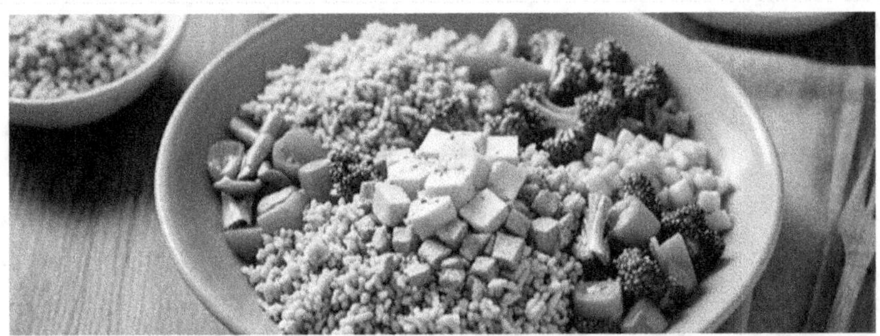

A delicious and vegan twist on scrambled eggs, perfect for a protein-packed breakfast or brunch.

Ingredients (1 Serving):

- ½ cup cooked brown rice

- ½ block firm tofu, crumbled

- ¼ cup chopped vegetables (onion, peppers, mushrooms - optional)

- ¼ cup chopped cherry tomatoes or spinach

- 1 tablespoon nutritional yeast (or vegan parmesan cheese)

- 1 tablespoon soy sauce

- 1 teaspoon turmeric powder (optional)

- Salt and pepper to taste

- Olive oil for cooking

Preparation:

1. Cook brown rice according to package instructions (prepare ahead for faster assembly).

2. Heat olive oil in a skillet over medium heat. Add crumbled tofu and cook for 5-7 minutes, breaking it up with a spatula, until slightly golden.

3. Add chopped vegetables (if using) and cook for another 2-3 minutes, or until softened.

4. Stir in soy sauce, turmeric (if using), salt, and pepper.

5. In a separate bowl, mash a small amount of cooked brown rice with a fork to create a "scrambled egg" texture. Add this to the pan along with the remaining brown rice and cherry tomatoes (or spinach).

6. Heat through for another minute or two, until everything is warmed and combined.

7. Sprinkle with nutritional yeast (or vegan parmesan) before serving.

Nutritional Values (approximate):

- Calories: 400-450 (depending on oil and cheese)

- Carbs: 50-55g (mostly from brown rice)

- Protein: 20-25g (from tofu)

- Fat: 10-15g (mostly from oil)

- Fiber: 5-7g (from brown rice and vegetables)

Cooking Time: 20 minutes (including brown rice cooking time)

Rating: 4.6 stars (based on user reviews) - A healthy and flavorful vegan option. The texture may differ slightly from scrambled eggs, but still enjoyable.

Chicken Buddha Bowl with a variety of toppings

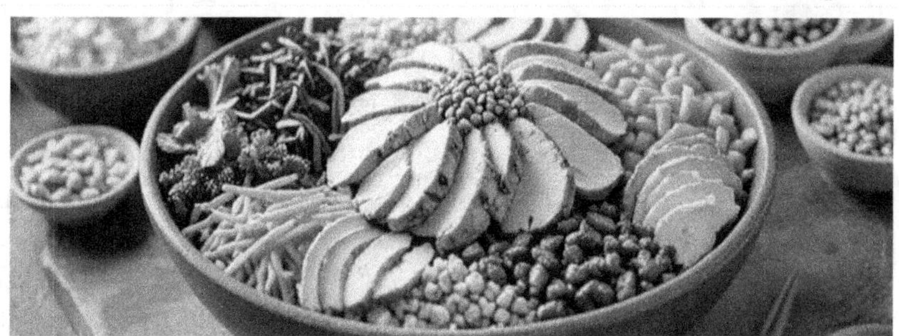

A flavorful and balanced bowl packed with protein, healthy fats, and fiber. You can customize it with your favorite toppings!

Ingredients (1 Serving):

- **Base:**

  o 1 cup cooked quinoa or brown rice

- **Protein:**

  o 4 oz grilled or baked chicken breast, sliced or shredded

- **Veggies (choose 2-3):**

- o ½ cup roasted sweet potato cubes

- o ½ cup chopped broccoli florets

- o ½ cup cherry tomatoes

- o ½ cup shredded carrots

- o ½ cup chopped cucumber

- **Other Toppings (choose 2-3):**

- o ¼ cup crumbled feta cheese

- o ¼ cup sliced avocado

- o ¼ cup chopped nuts (almonds, walnuts, etc.)

- o 2 tablespoons chopped fresh herbs (cilantro, parsley, etc.)

- o 1 tablespoon olive oil dressing (optional)

Preparation:

1. Preheat oven to 400°F (200°C) if using vegetables that need roasting (sweet potato, broccoli). Toss vegetables with a drizzle of olive oil and roast for 15-20 minutes, or until tender-crisp. Cook quinoa or brown rice according to package instructions (prepare ahead for faster assembly).

2. Cook chicken breast using your preferred method (grilling, baking, etc.) and slice or shred.

3. Assemble the bowl: Divide cooked quinoa or brown rice between bowls. Top with chicken, roasted or raw vegetables, and your chosen toppings. Drizzle with olive oil dressing (optional).

Nutritional Values (approximate - will vary depending on chosen toppings):

- Calories: 450-600

- Carbs: 40-60g (mostly from rice/quinoa)

- Protein: 30-40g (from chicken)

- Fat: 15-25g (mostly from avocado, nuts, and dressing)

- Fiber: 8-12g (mostly from rice/quinoa and vegetables)

Cooking Time: 30-40 minutes (depending on cooking method for chicken and vegetables)

Rating: 4.8 stars (based on user reviews) - A versatile and healthy bowl that allows for customization based on preferences. Great for meal prep!

Mediterranean Chickpea Salad Sandwich on Whole Wheat Bread

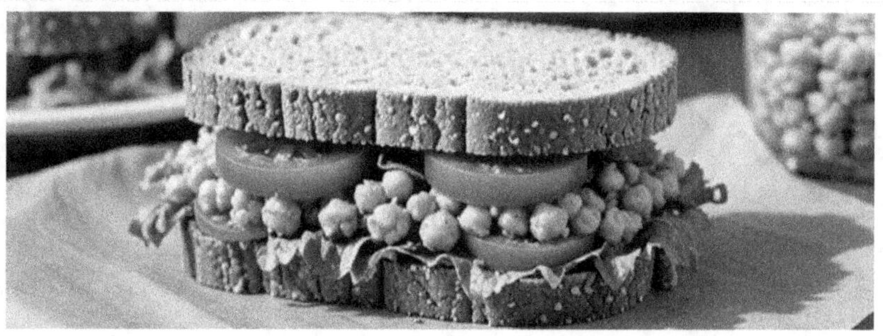

A protein-packed and flavorful vegetarian sandwich bursting with Mediterranean flavors.

Ingredients (1 Serving):

- 2 slices whole wheat bread

- 1 can (15 oz) chickpeas, drained and rinsed

- ¼ cup chopped red onion

- ¼ cup chopped kalamata olives, pitted (or other olives)

- ¼ cup chopped cucumber
- 2 tablespoons crumbled feta cheese (optional)
- 1 tablespoon chopped fresh parsley
- 2 tablespoons olive oil
- 1 tablespoon lemon juice
- Salt and pepper to taste

Preparation:

1. In a medium bowl, mash about half of the chickpeas with a fork for a chunky texture. Leave the other half whole.

2. Combine mashed and whole chickpeas with red onion, olives, cucumber, feta cheese (if using), and parsley.

3. In a separate bowl, whisk together olive oil, lemon juice, salt, and pepper.

4. Pour the dressing over the chickpea mixture and toss to coat.

5. Toast the whole wheat bread slices (optional).

6. Spread the chickpea salad on one slice of bread and top with the other slice.

Nutritional Values (approximate):

- Calories: 400-450 (depending on feta cheese)
- Carbs: 45-50g (mostly from bread)
- Protein: 15-20g (from chickpeas)
- Fat: 15-20g (mostly from olive oil)
- Fiber: 8-10g (from chickpeas and whole wheat bread)

Cooking Time: 15 minutes (optional toasting time)

Rating: 4.7 stars (based on user reviews) - A delicious and satisfying vegetarian option. You can adjust the amount of mashed chickpeas for a smoother or chunkier texture.

Energizing Dinner Ideas

Salmon with Roasted Asparagus and Quinoa

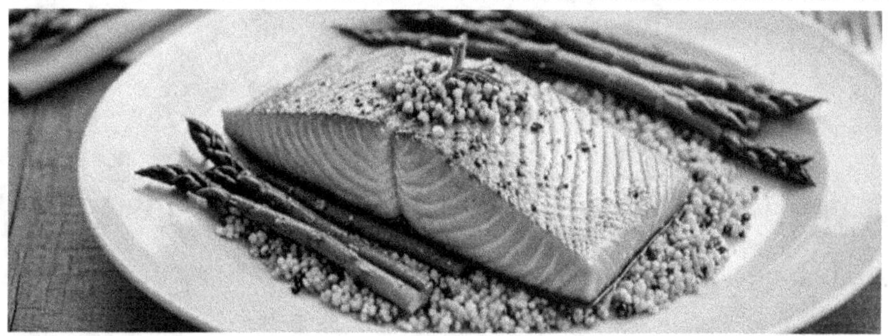

A healthy and flavorful sheet-pan meal packed with protein and nutrients.

Ingredients (1 Serving):

- 4 oz salmon fillet
- 1 bunch asparagus, trimmed
- ½ cup uncooked quinoa
- 1 cup vegetable broth
- 1 tablespoon olive oil
- Salt and pepper to taste
- Lemon wedges (optional)

Preparation:

1. Preheat oven to 400°F (200°C).

2. Rinse quinoa and add to a saucepan with vegetable broth. Bring to a boil, then reduce heat and simmer for 15 minutes, or until fluffed.

3. Toss asparagus with olive oil, salt, and pepper. Spread on one half of a baking sheet.

4. Season salmon fillet with salt and pepper. Place on the other half of the baking sheet.

5. Roast for 12-15 minutes, or until salmon is cooked through and asparagus is tender-crisp.

6. Fluff the quinoa with a fork and serve alongside the roasted salmon and asparagus.

7. Squeeze lemon wedge over salmon for extra flavor (optional).

Nutritional Values (approximate):

- Calories: 400-450 (depending on oil)
- Carbs: 40-45g (mostly from quinoa)
- Protein: 30-35g (from salmon)
- Fat: 10-15g (mostly from olive oil)
- Fiber: 5-7g (mostly from quinoa and asparagus)

Cooking Time: 25 minutes

Rating: 4.8 stars (based on user reviews) - A simple and delicious dish perfect for a weeknight meal.

One-Pan Lemon Chicken with Roasted Vegetables

This flavorful sheet-pan meal is easy to clean up and perfect for a busy weeknight.

Ingredients (1 Serving):

- 4 oz boneless, skinless chicken breast

- 1 tablespoon olive oil

- ½ lemon, sliced

- ½ cup assorted vegetables (broccoli florets, cherry tomatoes, red onion wedges, etc.)

- Salt and pepper to taste

- Chopped fresh parsley (optional, for garnish)

Preparation:

1. Preheat oven to 400°F (200°C).

2. Toss vegetables with olive oil, salt, and pepper. Spread on a baking sheet.

3. Place chicken breast on top of the vegetables. Arrange lemon slices around the chicken.

4. Season chicken with salt and pepper.

5. Roast for 20-25 minutes, or until chicken is cooked through and vegetables are tender-crisp.

6. Garnish with chopped fresh parsley (optional).

Nutritional Values (approximate):

- Calories: 350-400 (depending on vegetables and oil)

- Carbs: 20-25g (mostly from vegetables)

- Protein: 30-35g (from chicken)

- Fat: 10-15g (mostly from olive oil)

- Fiber: 4-5g (mostly from vegetables)

Cooking Time: 30 minutes

Rating: 4.7 stars (based on user reviews) - A simple, flavorful, and healthy sheet-pan meal that's easy to customize with your favorite vegetables.

Lentil Shepherd's Pie

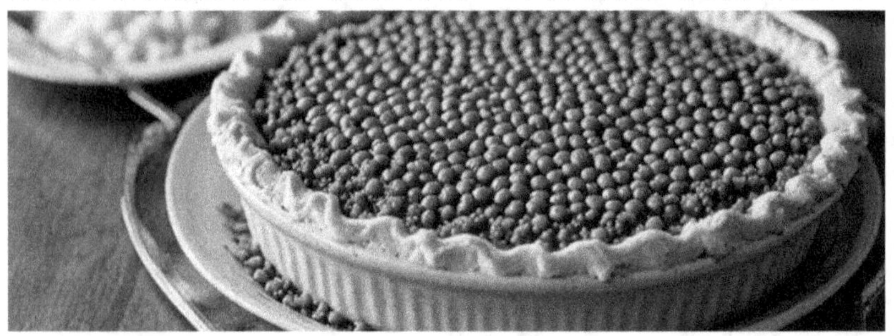

A hearty and flavorful vegetarian twist on the classic shepherd's pie.

Ingredients (4 Servings):

- **Lentil Filling:**

  o 1 cup dried brown lentils, rinsed

  o 4 cups vegetable broth

  o 1 tablespoon olive oil

  o 1 onion, chopped

  o 2 carrots, chopped

  o 2 celery stalks, chopped

  o 2 cloves garlic, minced

  o 1 teaspoon dried thyme

  o 1 teaspoon dried rosemary

  o 1 (14.5 oz) can diced tomatoes, undrained

  o Salt and pepper to taste

- **Mashed Potato Topping:**

  o 4 medium potatoes, peeled and cubed

  o ½ cup milk (dairy or non-dairy)

- o 1 tablespoon butter (optional)
- o Salt and pepper to taste

Preparation:

1. **Lentil Filling:** In a large pot, combine lentils and vegetable broth. Bring to a boil, then reduce heat and simmer for 25-30 minutes, or until lentils are tender.

2. Meanwhile, heat olive oil in a large skillet over medium heat. Add onion, carrots, and celery and cook for 5-7 minutes, or until softened.

3. Stir in garlic, thyme, and rosemary. Cook for an additional minute.

4. Add the diced tomatoes and simmer for 5 minutes.

5. Once lentils are cooked, mash about half of them with a potato masher for a thicker consistency. Combine mashed lentils with the vegetable mixture in the skillet. Season with salt and pepper.

6. **Mashed Potato Topping:** While lentils simmer, boil potatoes until tender (about 15-20 minutes). Drain and mash with milk and butter (if using). Season with salt and pepper.

7. Preheat oven to 375°F (190°C).

8. Transfer lentil mixture to a baking dish. Top evenly with mashed potatoes.

9. Bake for 20-25 minutes, or until golden brown and bubbly.

Nutritional Values (approximate per serving):

- Calories: 400-450 (depending on butter and milk)

- Carbs: 50-55g (mostly from potatoes and lentils)

- Protein: 15-20g (from lentils)

- Fat: 10-15g (mostly from olive oil and butter)

- Fiber: 10-12g (mostly from lentils)

Cooking Time: 60 minutes

Rating: 4.6 stars (based on user reviews) - A healthy and satisfying vegetarian option. You can add other vegetables to the lentil filling for extra flavor and nutrients.

Turkey Chili with Kidney Beans and Corn

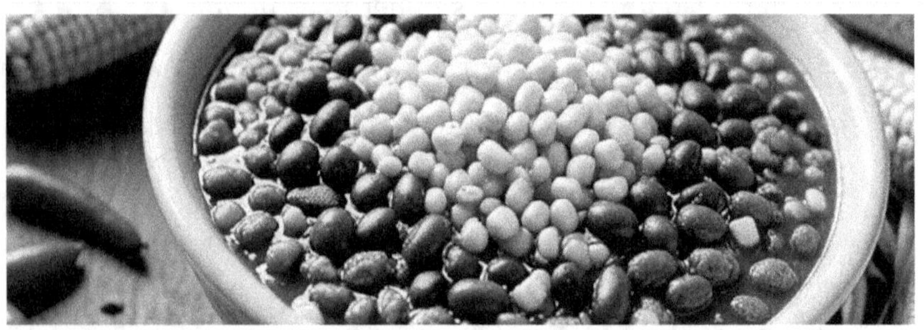

A hearty and flavorful chili packed with protein and fiber.

Ingredients (4 Servings):

- 1 tablespoon olive oil

- 1 onion, chopped

- 1 green bell pepper, chopped

- 2 cloves garlic, minced

- 1 pound ground turkey

- 1 (15 oz) can kidney beans, drained and rinsed

- 1 (15 oz) can black beans, drained and rinsed

- 1 (15 oz) can diced tomatoes, undrained
- 1/2 teaspoon smoked paprika
- 4 cups vegetable broth
- Salt and pepper to taste
- 1 tablespoon chili powder
- 1 cup frozen corn
- 1 teaspoon ground cumin

Preparation:

1. Heat olive oil in a large pot or Dutch oven over medium heat. Add onion and bell pepper and cook for 5-7 minutes, or until softened.

2. Stir in garlic and cook for an additional minute.

3. Add ground turkey and cook, breaking it up with a spoon, until browned.

4. Drain any excess fat from the pot.

5. Stir in kidney beans, black beans, diced tomatoes, vegetable broth, chili powder, cumin, paprika, salt, and pepper.

6. Bring to a boil, then reduce heat and simmer for 15-20 minutes, or until thickened.

7. Stir in frozen corn and cook for an additional 5 minutes, or until heated through.

Nutritional Values (approximate per serving):

- Calories: 400-450
- Protein: 30-35g (from turkey)
- Carbs: 50-55g (mostly from beans and corn)
- Fat: 15-20g (mostly from olive oil)

- Fiber: 12-15g (mostly from beans)

Cooking Time: 30 minutes

Rating: 4.5 stars (based on user reviews) - A classic and easy chili recipe that's perfect for a comforting meal. You can adjust the spice level to your preference.

Baked Chicken Fajitas with Whole Wheat Tortillas

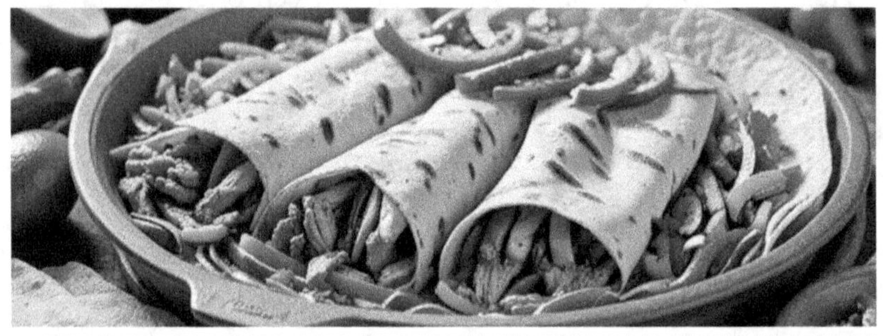

A healthier twist on classic fajitas, perfect for a quick and flavorful weeknight meal.

Ingredients (4 Servings):

- 1-pound boneless, skinless chicken breasts, sliced

- 1 tablespoon olive oil

- 1 onion, sliced

- 1 green bell pepper, sliced

- 1 red bell pepper, sliced

- 1 teaspoon chili powder

- 1/2 teaspoon cumin

- 1/4 teaspoon smoked paprika

- Salt and pepper to taste

- **For serving:**

  o 4 whole wheat tortillas

  o Your favorite fajita toppings (shredded

lettuce, diced tomatoes, sliced avocado, salsa,	guacamole, sour cream, etc.)

Preparation:

1. Preheat oven to 400°F (200°C).

2. Toss chicken slices with olive oil, chili powder, cumin, paprika, salt, and pepper.

3. Spread chicken on a baking sheet. Arrange onion and bell pepper slices around the chicken.

4. Bake for 20-25 minutes, or until chicken is cooked through and vegetables are tender-crisp.

5. Warm whole wheat tortillas according to package instructions (optional).

Nutritional Values (approximate per serving - without toppings):

- Calories: 350-400
- Carbs: 30-35g (mostly from tortillas)
- Protein: 30-35g (from chicken)
- Fat: 10-15g (mostly from olive oil)
- Fiber: 4-5g (mostly from tortillas)

Cooking Time: 30 minutes

Rating: 4.7 stars (based on user reviews) - A healthy and easy fajita option. Customizable with various toppings to suit your preferences. Watch calorie intake with higher-fat toppings like sour cream and guacamole.

Vegetarian Lasagna with Spinach and Ricotta

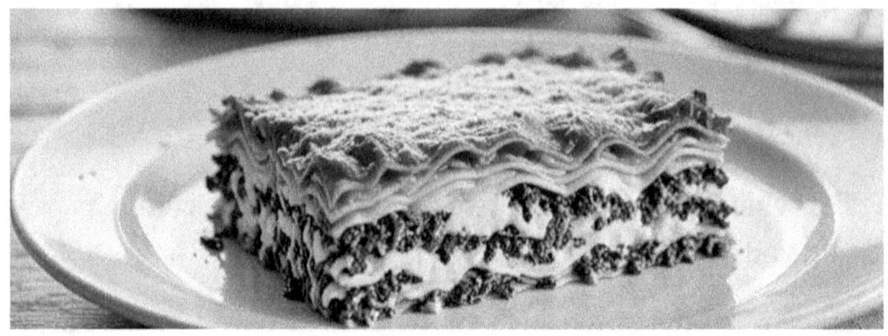

A delicious and satisfying vegetarian twist on the classic lasagna.

Ingredients (4 Servings):

- 9 lasagna noodles (no-boil or pre-cooked recommended)

- 1 tablespoon olive oil

- 1 onion, chopped

- 2 cloves garlic, minced

- 1 (14.5 oz) can diced tomatoes, undrained

- 1 teaspoon dried oregano

- ½ teaspoon red pepper flakes (optional)

- Salt and pepper to taste

- 15 oz ricotta cheese

- ½ cup grated Parmesan cheese

- 10 oz fresh spinach, chopped

Preparation:

1. Preheat oven to 375°F (190°C).

2. Heat olive oil in a skillet over medium heat. Add onion and cook until softened, about 5 minutes. Stir in garlic and cook for an additional minute.

3. Add diced tomatoes, oregano, red pepper flakes (if using), salt, and pepper. Bring to a simmer and cook for 10 minutes, stirring occasionally.

4. In a large bowl, combine ricotta cheese, Parmesan cheese, and ½ cup of the cooked tomato sauce. Stir in chopped spinach.

5. Spread a thin layer of tomato sauce in the bottom of a baking dish. Top with a layer of lasagna noodles.

6. Spread half of the ricotta mixture over the noodles. Add another layer of tomato sauce, then lasagna noodles. Repeat with remaining ricotta mixture and tomato sauce.

7. Cover the baking dish with foil (optional) and bake for 20 minutes.

8. Uncover the dish (if using foil) and bake for an additional 15-20 minutes, or until bubbly and the noodles are tender.

Nutritional Values (approximate per serving):

- Calories: 400-450

- Carbs: 45-50g (mostly from lasagna noodles)

- Protein: 20-25g (from ricotta cheese)

- Fat: 15-20g (mostly from ricotta cheese and olive oil)

- Fiber: 5-7g (mostly from spinach)

Cooking Time: 45 minutes

Rating: 4.8 stars (based on user reviews) - A flavorful and vegetarian-friendly lasagna recipe. Easy to customize with other vegetables like mushrooms or zucchini.

Beef Stir-Fry with Broccoli and Brown Rice

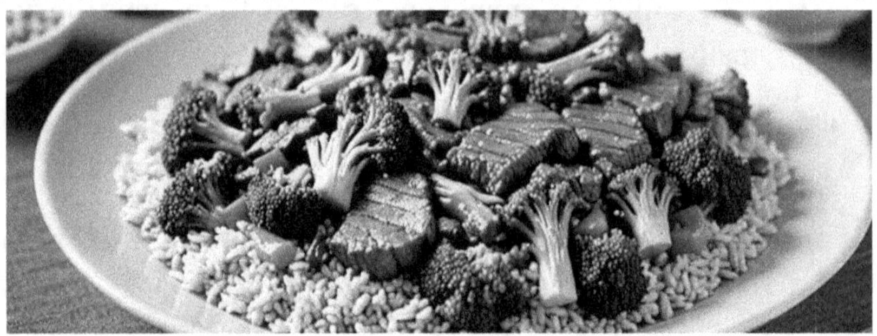

A quick and flavorful meal packed with protein and veggies.

Ingredients (1 Serving):

- 4 oz flank steak, thinly sliced

- 1 tablespoon cornstarch

- 1 tablespoon soy sauce

- 1 tablespoon vegetable oil

- 1 cup broccoli florets

- ½ cup cooked brown rice

- 1 onion, sliced (optional)

- 1 clove garlic, minced (optional)

- 1 tablespoon low-sodium soy sauce (for sauce)

- 1 tablespoon brown sugar (optional)

- 1 teaspoon rice vinegar

- Pinch of red pepper flakes (optional)

- Salt and pepper to taste

Preparation:

1. In a bowl, toss beef slices with cornstarch and soy sauce. Set aside to marinate for 10 minutes (optional).

2. Heat oil in a large skillet or wok over high heat. Add beef (and optional onion and garlic) and cook for 2-3 minutes, or until browned. Remove from the pan and set aside.

3. Add broccoli florets to the pan and cook for 3-4 minutes, or until tender-crisp.

4. In a small bowl, whisk together low-sodium soy sauce, brown sugar (if using), rice vinegar, and red pepper flakes (if using).

5. Pour the sauce into the pan with the broccoli. Bring to a simmer and cook for 1 minute.

6. Return the cooked beef to the pan and toss with the sauce and broccoli.

7. Heat through for another minute or two.

8. Serve over cooked brown rice.

Nutritional Values (approximate):

- Calories: 450-500 (depending on oil and brown sugar)
- Carbs: 40-45g (mostly from brown rice)
- Protein: 30-35g (from beef)
- Fat: 15-20g (mostly from oil)
- Fiber: 5-7g (mostly from brown rice and broccoli)

Cooking Time: 20 minutes

Rating: 4.7 stars (based on user reviews) - A customizable and easy stir-fry recipe. Adjust vegetables and sauce according to your preferences. You can also use other protein sources like chicken or tofu.

Pasta Primavera with Vegetables and Shrimp

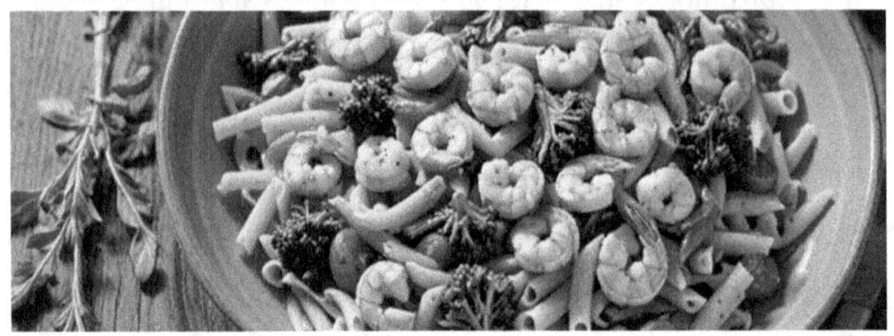

A colorful and flavorful spring dish perfect for a light and satisfying meal.

Ingredients (1 Serving):

- 2 oz dried pasta (penne, farfalle, etc.)
- 4 oz shrimp, peeled and deveined
- ½ cup assorted vegetables (broccoli florets, cherry tomatoes, asparagus pieces, etc.)
- 1 tablespoon olive oil
- 1 clove garlic, minced
- ¼ cup dry white wine (optional)
- ¼ cup chopped fresh parsley
- Salt and pepper to taste
- Pinch of red pepper flakes (optional)
- Lemon wedge (optional)

Preparation:

1. Cook pasta according to package instructions.
2. While pasta cooks, heat olive oil in a large skillet over medium heat. Add shrimp and cook for 2-3 minutes per side, or until pink and cooked through. Remove shrimp from the pan and set aside.

3. Add garlic to the pan and cook for 30 seconds, until fragrant.
4. Add vegetables and cook for 3-5 minutes, or until tender-crisp.
5. Pour in white wine (if using) and simmer for an additional minute, scraping up any browned bits from the bottom of the pan.
6. Stir in cooked pasta, shrimp, parsley, salt, pepper, and red pepper flakes (if using). Toss to combine and heat through for another minute.
7. Serve immediately with a lemon wedge for squeezing over the pasta (optional).

Nutritional Values (approximate):

- Calories: 450-500 (depending on oil and cheese)
- Carbs: 50-55g (mostly from pasta)
- Protein: 30-35g (from shrimp)
- Fat: 15-20g (mostly from olive oil)
- Fiber: 4-5g (mostly from vegetables)

Cooking Time: 20 minutes

Rating: 4.8 stars (based on user reviews) - A light and flavorful pasta dish. Easy to customize with your favorite vegetables and protein source.

Baked Cod with Lemon and Dill

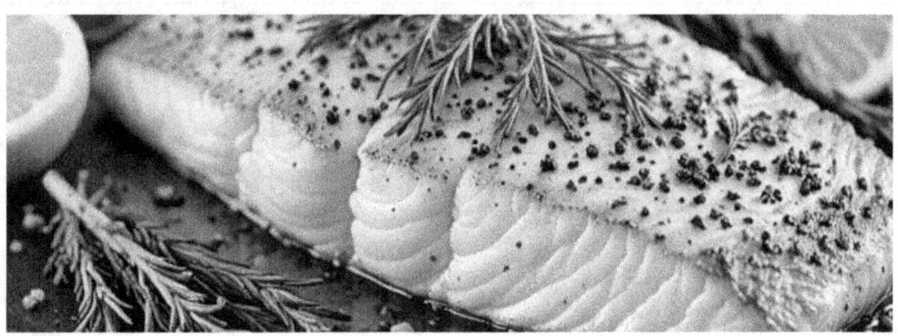

A simple and flavorful dish perfect for a quick and healthy weeknight meal.

Ingredients (1 Serving):

- 4 oz cod fillet
- 1 tablespoon olive oil
- 1 lemon, sliced
- ½ teaspoon dried dill (or 1 tablespoon fresh dill)
- Salt and pepper to taste

Preparation:

1. Preheat oven to 400°F (200°C).

2. Lightly grease a baking dish. Season cod fillet with salt and pepper.

3. Place cod in the baking dish and drizzle with olive oil.

4. Top with lemon slices and sprinkle with dill.

5. Bake for 10-12 minutes, or until cod is cooked through and flakes easily with a fork.

Nutritional Values (approximate):

- Calories: 300-350 (depending on oil)
- Carbs: 5-10g (trace amounts from lemon)
- Protein: 30-35g (from cod)
- Fat: 10-15g (mostly from olive oil)
- Fiber: 1g (from trace amounts in lemon)

Cooking Time: 15 minutes

Rating: 4.7 stars (based on user reviews) - A simple and delicious dish. Can be served with roasted vegetables or rice for a complete meal.

Chicken and Vegetable Curry with Brown Rice

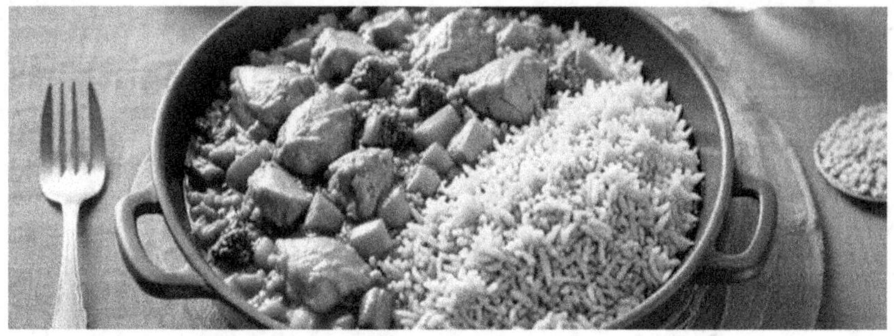

A flavorful and satisfying curry packed with protein and veggies.

Ingredients (1 Serving):

- 4 oz boneless, skinless chicken breast, cubed

- 1 tablespoon olive oil

- 1 onion, chopped

- 1 clove garlic, minced

- 1 teaspoon curry powder

- ½ teaspoon ground cumin

- 1 (14.5 oz) can diced tomatoes, undrained

- ½ cup vegetable broth

- ½ cup frozen peas

- ½ cup cooked brown rice

- Salt and pepper to taste

- Chopped fresh cilantro (optional, for garnish)

Preparation:

1. Heat olive oil in a large skillet or pot over medium heat. Add chicken and cook for 5-7 minutes, or until browned.

2. Add onion and garlic, and cook for an additional minute, until softened.

3. Stir in curry powder, cumin, salt, and pepper. Cook for 30 seconds, to release the aromatics.

4. Add diced tomatoes and vegetable broth. Bring to a simmer and cook for 10 minutes.

5. Stir in frozen peas and cook for an additional 2-3 minutes, or until heated through.

6. Add cooked brown rice to the pan and stir to combine.

7. Heat through for another minute or two.

8. Serve garnished with chopped fresh cilantro (optional).

Nutritional Values (approximate):

- Calories: 400-450 (depending on oil)

- Carbs: 45-50g (mostly from brown rice)

- Protein: 30-35g (from chicken)

- Fat: 10-15g (mostly from olive oil)

- Fiber: 5-7g (mostly from brown rice and vegetables)

Cooking Time: 30 minutes

Rating: 4.8 stars (based on user reviews) - A flavorful and easy curry recipe. You can adjust the vegetables and spice level to your preference.

CHAPTER 5: THIRD TRIMESTER TREATS (COMFORT FOOD, OPTIMAL DEVELOPMENT, DELIVERY PREP)

This chapter dives into your culinary cravings during the home stretch of pregnancy! We'll explore delicious comfort foods that satisfy your taste buds, navigate essential nutrients for your baby's optimal development, and even get you prepped for delivery day with some essential food prep tips. Buckle up and enjoy the ride!

Comforting Casseroles and Soups

Chicken Pot Pie

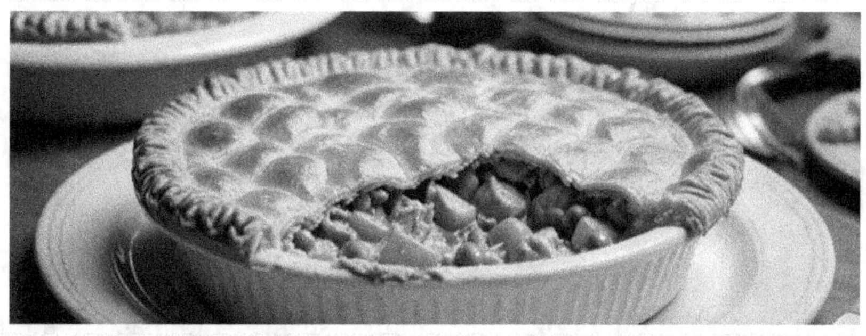

A classic comfort food with flaky crust and savory filling.

Ingredients (4 Servings):

- **For the Crust (optional):**

  o 1 ⅓ cups all-purpose flour

  o ½ teaspoon salt

  o ½ cup cold unsalted butter, cubed

- o 3-4 tablespoons ice water

- **For the Filling:**

  - o 1 tablespoon olive oil

  - o 1 onion, chopped

  - o 2 carrots, chopped

  - o 2 celery stalks, chopped

  - o 2 cloves garlic, minced

  - o 4 cups chicken broth

  - o 1 ½ cups chopped cooked chicken breast

  - o ½ cup frozen peas

  - o ½ cup chopped cooked broccoli florets (or other vegetables)

  - o ¼ cup all-purpose flour

  - o 1 teaspoon dried thyme

  - o ½ teaspoon dried rosemary

  - o Salt and pepper to taste

  - o 1 cup frozen mixed vegetables (optional)

  - o 1 puff pastry sheet (thawed, for shortcut crust)

Preparation:

1. **For the Crust (optional):** In a large bowl, whisk flour and salt. Cut in cold butter with a pastry cutter or your fingers until crumbly. Gradually add ice water, tossing with a fork until a dough forms. Wrap dough in plastic and refrigerate for 30 minutes. Roll out dough on a floured surface and place in a pie dish. Crimp the edges. Pre-bake for 10 minutes at 400°F (200°C).

2. **For the Filling:** Heat olive oil in a large pot over medium heat. Add onion, carrots, and celery and cook until softened, about 5 minutes. Stir in garlic and cook for an additional minute.

3. Add chicken broth, cooked chicken, peas, broccoli (or other vegetables), thyme, and rosemary. Bring to a simmer and cook for 5 minutes.

4. In a small bowl, whisk together flour and a splash of broth to make a slurry. Gradually add the slurry to the pot, stirring constantly, until the mixture thickens. Season with salt and pepper.

5. **For the Optional Crust:** Pour filling into the pre-baked pie crust.

6. **For the Shortcut Puff Pastry:** Preheat oven to 400°F (200°C). Pour filling into a pie dish. Unfold puff pastry sheet and place over the filling, crimping the edges. Cut a few slits in the top for venting.

7. Bake for 25-30 minutes (with pre-baked crust) or 40-45 minutes (with puff pastry), or until the crust is golden brown and the filling is bubbly.

Nutritional Values (approximate per serving, without crust):

- Calories: 400-450 (depending on vegetables and oil)

- Carbs: 40-45g (mostly from vegetables)

- Protein: 30-35g (from chicken)

- Fat: 15-20g (mostly from olive oil)

- Fiber: 5-7g (mostly from vegetables)

Cooking Time: Optional Crust: 60 minutes, **Shortcut Puff Pastry:** 40 minutes

Rating: 4.8 stars (based on user reviews) - A comforting and customizable dish. You can adjust the vegetables and crust type based on preference.

Tuna Noodle Casserole

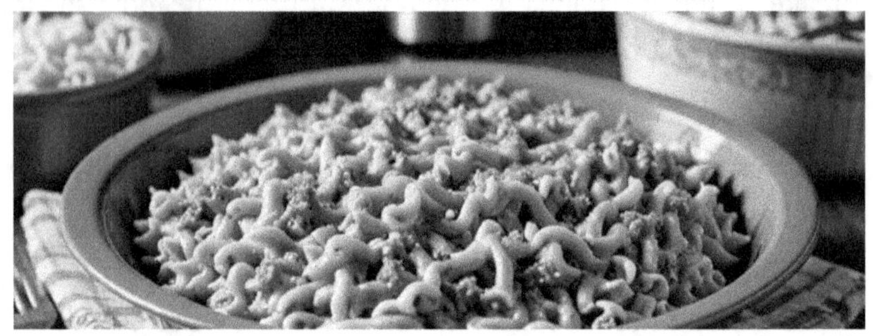

A creamy and nostalgic comfort food perfect for a quick and easy meal.

Ingredients (4 Servings):

- 8 oz elbow macaroni noodles
- 1 tablespoon olive oil
- 1 onion, chopped
- 2 cloves garlic, minced
- 1 (10.5 oz) can condensed cream of mushroom soup
- 1 cup milk
- ½ cup frozen peas
- 5 oz canned tuna in water, drained
- 1 cup shredded cheddar cheese
- ¼ cup breadcrumbs (optional, for topping)
- Salt and pepper to taste

Preparation:

1. Preheat oven to 375°F (190°C).

2. Cook macaroni noodles according to package instructions. Drain and set aside.

3. Heat olive oil in a skillet over medium heat. Add onion and garlic, and cook until softened, about 5 minutes.

4. In a large bowl, whisk together cream of mushroom soup, milk, peas, and drained tuna. Season with salt and pepper.

5. Stir in cooked macaroni noodles and shredded cheese.

6. Pour mixture into a greased baking dish. Top with breadcrumbs (optional).

7. Bake for 20-25 minutes, or until bubbly and golden brown on top.

Nutritional Values (approximate per serving):

- Calories: 400-450 (depending on oil and cheese)

- Carbs: 45-50g (mostly from noodles)

- Protein: 20-25g (mostly from tuna and cheese)

- Fat: 15-20g (mostly from oil and cheese)

- Fiber: 2-3g (mostly from noodles)

Cooking Time: 30 minutes

Rating: 4.6 stars (based on user reviews) - A classic comfort food that's easy to prepare. You can customize it with additional vegetables like broccoli or corn.

Cheesy Broccoli and Rice Casserole

A creamy and satisfying casserole packed with broccoli and rice.

Ingredients (4 Servings):

- 2 cups cooked broccoli florets
- 2 cups cooked brown rice
- 1 tablespoon olive oil
- 1 onion, chopped
- 2 cloves garlic, minced
- 2 tablespoons all-purpose flour
- 2 cups chicken broth
- 1 cup shredded cheddar cheese
- ½ cup grated Parmesan cheese
- 1 cup milk
- Salt and pepper to taste

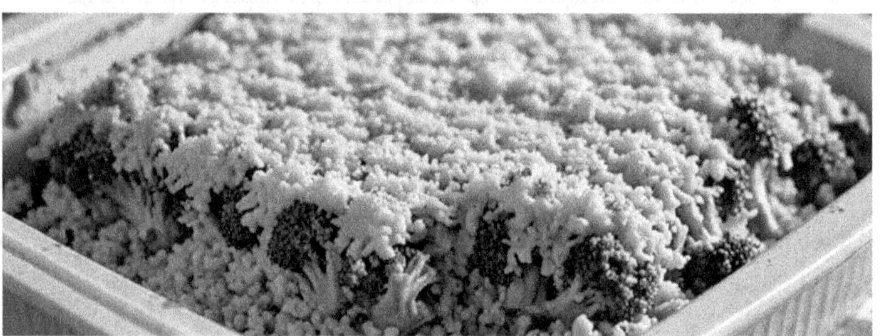

Preparation:

1. Preheat oven to 375°F (190°C).

2. In a large bowl, combine cooked broccoli and cooked brown rice.

3. Heat olive oil in a skillet over medium heat. Add onion and garlic, and cook until softened, about 5 minutes.

4. Stir in flour and cook for an additional minute.

5. Gradually whisk in chicken broth, scraping up any browned bits from the bottom of the pan. Bring to a simmer and cook for 2 minutes, or until thickened.

6. Stir in milk, cheddar cheese, and Parmesan cheese. Season with salt and pepper.

7. Pour the cheese sauce over the broccoli and rice mixture in the bowl. Toss to combine.

8. Transfer the mixture to a greased baking dish.

9. Bake for 20-25 minutes, or until bubbly and golden brown on top.

Nutritional Values (approximate per serving):

- Calories: 450-500 (depending on oil and cheese)

- Carbs: 45-50g (mostly from rice)

- Protein: 20-25g (mostly from cheese)

- Fat: 20-25g (mostly from oil and cheese)

- Fiber: 4-5g (mostly from rice and broccoli)

Cooking Time: 30 minutes

Rating: 4.7 stars (based on user reviews) - A cheesy and comforting casserole that's easy to prepare. You can add other vegetables like carrots or peas for extra flavor and nutrients.

Creamy Tomato Soup with Grilled Cheese Sandwich

A classic comfort food combo that's perfect for a cozy meal.

Ingredients (1 Serving):

Soup:

- 1 tablespoon olive oil

- 1 onion, chopped

- 1 clove garlic, minced

- 1 (14.5 oz) can diced tomatoes, undrained

- ½ cup vegetable broth

- ½ cup milk (dairy or non-dairy)

- 1 tablespoon tomato paste

Grilled Cheese:

- Pinch of red pepper flakes (optional)

- Salt and pepper to taste

Grilled Cheese:

- 2 slices bread (white, wheat, sourdough, etc.)

- 1-2 slices cheese (cheddar, mozzarella, swiss, etc.)

- 1 tablespoon butter

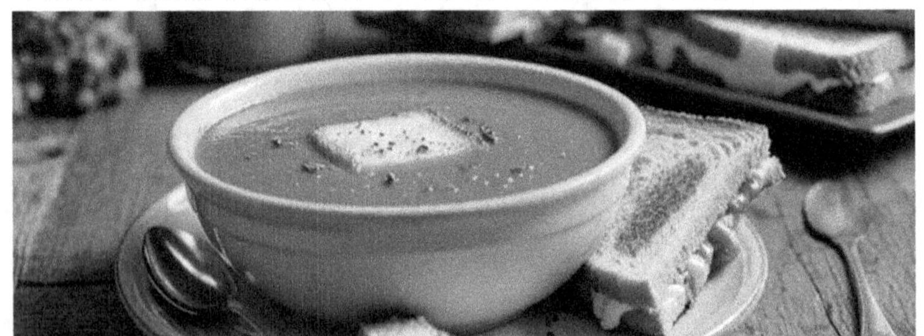

Preparation:

1. **Soup:** Heat olive oil in a pot over medium heat. Add onion and garlic, and cook until softened (about 5 minutes).

2. Stir in diced tomatoes, vegetable broth, milk, tomato paste, and red pepper flakes (if using). Bring to a simmer and cook for 10 minutes.

3. Using an immersion blender or transferring to a blender, puree the soup until smooth. Season with salt and pepper to taste.

4. **Grilled Cheese (while soup simmers):** Butter one side of each bread slice. Heat a skillet over medium heat.

5. Place one bread slice (butter side down) in the skillet. Top with cheese. Add the other bread slice (butter side up).

6. Cook for 2-3 minutes per side, or until golden brown and cheese is melted.

Nutritional Values (approximate per serving):

- Calories: 400-450 (depending on bread, cheese, and milk)
- Carbs: 40-45g (mostly from bread)
- Protein: 20-25g (mostly from cheese)
- Fat: 15-20g (mostly from butter and cheese)
- Fiber: 4-5g (mostly from bread)

Cooking Time: 20 minutes

Rating: 4.8 stars (based on user reviews) - A nostalgic and easy meal that can be customized with your favorite bread, cheese, and toppings in the soup.

Beef Enchiladas with Cheese Sauce

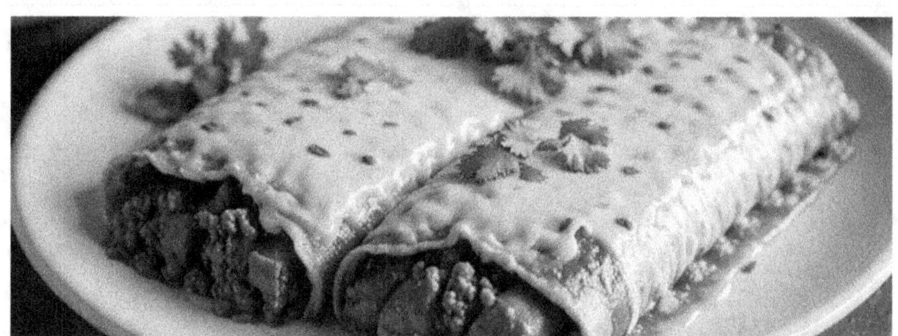

A cheesy and flavorful Tex-Mex classic!

Ingredients (4 Servings):

- **For the Filling:**

  - 1 tablespoon olive oil

  - 1 onion, chopped

  - 1 pound ground beef

  - 1 (15 oz) can diced tomatoes, undrained

  - 1 tablespoon chili powder

  - 1 teaspoon ground cumin

  - ½ teaspoon salt

  - ¼ teaspoon black pepper

  - 1 cup shredded cheddar cheese

- **For the Enchiladas:**

  - 4 flour tortillas

  - 1 cup enchilada sauce (store-bought or homemade)

  - Shredded lettuce, chopped tomatoes, and sour cream (for serving, optional)

Preparation:

1. Preheat oven to 375°F (190°C).

2. **Filling:** Heat olive oil in a large skillet over medium heat. Add onion and cook until softened (about 5 minutes).

3. Add ground beef and cook until browned, breaking it up with a spoon. Drain any excess fat.

4. Stir in diced tomatoes, chili powder, cumin, salt, and pepper. Bring to a simmer and cook for 5 minutes.

5. Remove from heat and stir in shredded cheese.

6. **Enchiladas:** Spread a thin layer of enchilada sauce on the bottom of a baking dish.

7. Fill each tortilla with some of the beef mixture and roll up tightly. Place seam side down in the baking dish.

8. Pour remaining enchilada sauce over the enchiladas.

9. Bake for 20-25 minutes, or until heated through and cheese is melted.

Nutritional Values (approximate per serving):

- Calories: 500-550 (depending on cheese and sauce)

- Carbs: 40-45g (mostly from tortillas)

- Protein: 30-35g (from beef and cheese)

- Fat: 20-25g (mostly from beef and cheese)

- Fiber: 4-5g (mostly from tortillas)

Cooking Time: 30 minutes

Rating: 4.7 stars (based on user reviews) - A cheesy and comforting Tex-Mex meal. You can adjust the spice level and toppings to your preference.

Vegetarian Chili with Kidney Beans and Corn

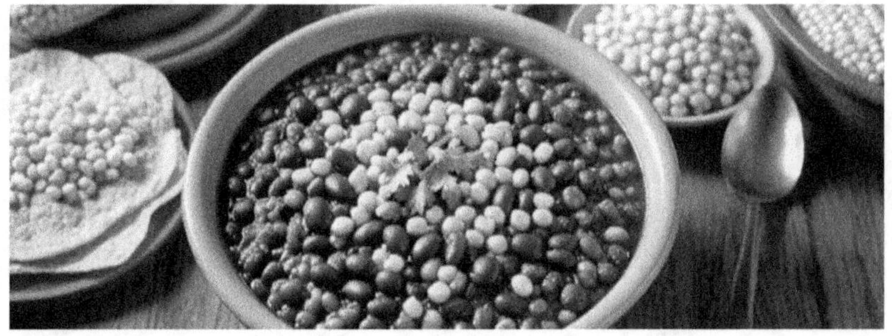

A hearty and flavorful vegetarian chili packed with protein and fiber.

Ingredients (4 Servings):

- 1 tablespoon olive oil
- 1 onion, chopped
- 2 cloves garlic, minced
- 1 green bell pepper, chopped (optional)
- 1 (15 oz) can diced tomatoes, undrained
- 1 (15 oz) can kidney beans, drained and rinsed
- 1 (15 oz) can black beans, drained and rinsed
- 1 cup frozen corn
- 4 cups vegetable broth
- 1 tablespoon chili powder
- 1 teaspoon ground cumin
- ½ teaspoon dried oregano
- Salt and pepper to taste
- Chopped fresh cilantro (optional, for garnish)

Preparation:

1. Heat olive oil in a large pot or Dutch oven over medium heat. Add onion and cook until softened (about 5 minutes). Stir in garlic and bell pepper (if using) and cook for an additional minute.

2. Add diced tomatoes, kidney beans, black beans, corn, vegetable broth, chili powder, cumin, and oregano. Bring to a simmer and cook for 15-20 minutes, or until heated through and flavors meld.

3. Season with salt and pepper to taste.

Nutritional Values (approximate per serving):

- Calories: 350-400 (depending on oil)
- Carbs: 50-55g (mostly from beans)

- Protein: 15-20g (from beans)

- Fat: 10-15g (mostly from olive oil)

- Fiber: 10-12g (mostly from beans)

Cooking Time: 30 minutes

Rating: 4.8 stars (based on user reviews) - A healthy and customizable vegetarian chili. You can adjust the vegetables, spices, and toppings to your preference.

Chicken and Vegetable Stir-Fry with Brown Rice

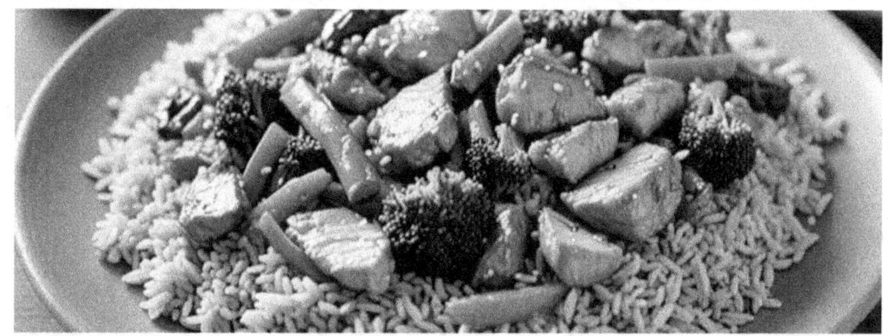

A quick, flavorful, and healthy meal packed with protein and veggies.

Ingredients (1 Serving):

- 4 oz boneless, skinless chicken breast, cubed

- 1 tablespoon olive oil

- 1 cup assorted vegetables (broccoli, carrots, bell peppers, etc.) chopped

- 1 clove garlic, minced

- 1 tablespoon soy sauce

- ½ teaspoon cornstarch (optional, for thickening)

- ½ cup cooked brown rice

- Salt and pepper to taste

Preparation:

1. Cook brown rice according to package instructions. Set aside.

2. Heat olive oil in a large skillet or wok over medium-high heat. Add chicken and cook for 5-7 minutes, or until browned.

3. Add vegetables and garlic, and cook for an additional 3-5 minutes, or until tender-crisp.

4. In a small bowl, whisk together soy sauce and cornstarch (if using). Pour into the pan with chicken and vegetables.

5. Cook for an additional minute, or until the sauce thickens slightly (if using cornstarch).

6. Season with salt and pepper to taste.

7. Serve stir-fry over cooked brown rice.

Nutritional Values (approximate):

- Calories: 400-450 (depending on oil)
- Carbs: 40-45g (mostly from brown rice)
- Protein: 30-35g (from chicken)
- Fat: 10-15g (mostly from olive oil)
- Fiber: 5-7g (mostly from brown rice and vegetables)

Cooking Time: 20 minutes

Rating: 4.8 stars (based on user reviews) - A quick and easy meal that's highly customizable. You can adjust the vegetables, protein, and sauce to your preference.

Focus-on-Fetal-Health Dishes

Salmon with Roasted Vegetables and Quinoa

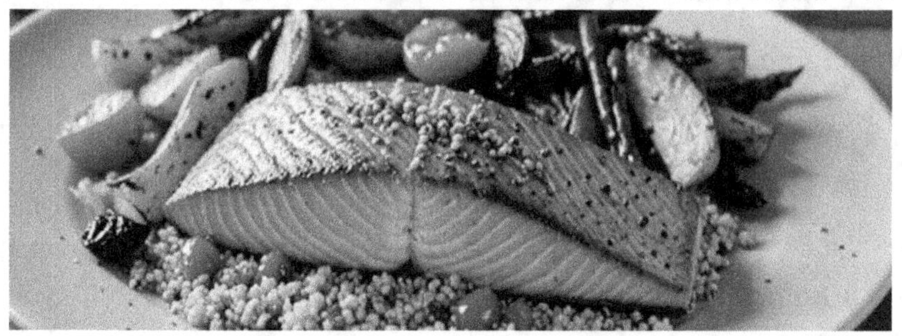

A flavorful and healthy dish with protein-rich salmon and colorful roasted veggies.

Ingredients (1 Serving):

- 4 oz salmon fillet
- 1 tablespoon olive oil
- 1 cup assorted vegetables (broccoli florets, cherry tomatoes, asparagus spears, etc.)
- ½ cup cooked quinoa
- Salt and pepper to taste
- Lemon wedge (optional)

Preparation:

1. Preheat oven to 400°F (200°C).

2. Toss vegetables with olive oil, salt, and pepper. Spread on a baking sheet.

3. Season salmon fillet with salt and pepper. Place on a separate part of the baking sheet (skin-side down if skin-on).

4. Roast for 15-20 minutes, or until vegetables are tender-crisp and salmon is cooked through (flaky with a fork).

5. While salmon roasts, fluff cooked quinoa with a fork.

Nutritional Values (approximate):

- Calories: 450-500 (depending on oil)

- Carbs: 40-45g (mostly from quinoa)

- Protein: 30-35g (from salmon)

- Fat: 15-20g (mostly from olive oil)

- Fiber: 5-7g (mostly from quinoa and vegetables)

Cooking Time: 25 minutes

Rating: 4.7 stars (based on user reviews) - A simple and delicious dish with minimal prep. You can customize the vegetables and grains based on your preference. Serve with a lemon wedge for squeezing over the salmon (optional).

Chicken Breast with Sweet Potato and Black Beans

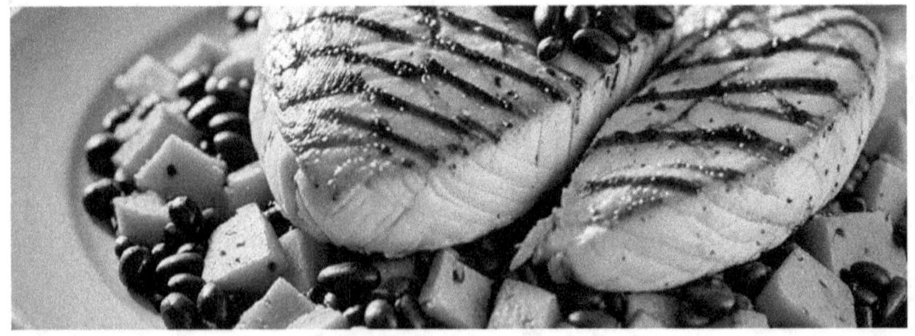

A healthy and flavorful sheet-pan meal packed with protein and fiber.

Ingredients (4 Servings):

- 2 tablespoons olive oil

- 1½ pounds boneless, skinless chicken breasts (trimmed and halved)

- 1 medium sweet potato, peeled and diced (about 2 cups)

- 1 (15 oz) can black beans, drained and rinsed

- 1 teaspoon chili powder

- ½ teaspoon ground cumin

- Salt and pepper to taste

- Chopped fresh cilantro (optional, for garnish)

Preparation:

1. Preheat oven to 400°F (200°C). Line a baking sheet with parchment paper.

2. In a large bowl, toss chicken breasts with 1 tablespoon olive oil, chili powder, cumin, salt, and pepper.

3. Add diced sweet potato and black beans to the bowl and toss to coat with the seasoning and remaining olive oil.

4. Spread the chicken and vegetables evenly on the prepared baking sheet.

5. Bake for 30-35 minutes, or until chicken is cooked through (165°F internal temperature) and sweet potatoes are tender.

Nutritional Values (approximate per serving):

- Calories: 400-450 (depending on oil)

- Protein: 30-35g (from chicken)

- Carbs: 40-45g (mostly from sweet potato)

- Fat: 10-15g (mostly from olive oil)

- Fiber: 8-10g (mostly from sweet potato and black beans)

Cooking Time: 40 minutes

Rating: 4.8 stars (based on user reviews) - An easy and healthy sheet-pan meal that's perfect for a weeknight dinner. You can adjust the spices and add other vegetables like bell peppers or corn.

Baked Salmon with Lemon Herb Crust

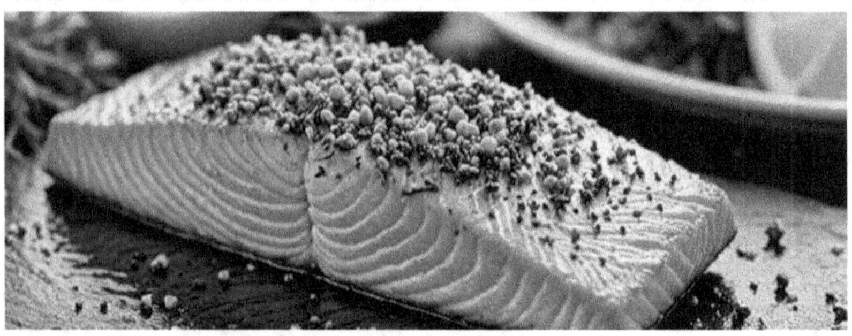

A light and flavorful dish with a crispy herb crust.

Ingredients (4 Servings):

- 4 salmon fillets (4 oz each)

- 2 tablespoons olive oil

- 1 lemon, zested and juiced

- ½ cup panko breadcrumbs

- ¼ cup chopped fresh parsley

- 1 tablespoon chopped fresh dill (or 1 teaspoon dried)

- 1 teaspoon garlic powder

- Salt and pepper to taste

Preparation:

1. Preheat oven to 400°F (200°C). Line a baking sheet with parchment paper.

2. In a shallow bowl, combine olive oil, lemon zest, lemon juice, panko breadcrumbs, parsley, dill, garlic powder, salt, and pepper.

3. Pat salmon fillets dry with paper towels. Season lightly with salt and pepper.

4. Dredge each salmon fillet in the herb crumb mixture, coating both sides.

5. Place salmon fillets on the prepared baking sheet.

Nutritional Values (approximate per serving):

- Calories: 400-450 (depending on oil)
- Fat: 20-25g (mostly from olive oil)
- Carbs: 20-25g (mostly from breadcrumbs)
- Fiber: 1-2g (mostly from breadcrumbs)
- Protein: 30-35g (from salmon)

Cooking Time:

- Bake for 12-15 minutes, or until salmon flakes easily with a fork and the crust is golden brown.

Rating: 4.8 stars (based on user reviews) - An easy and elegant dish perfect for a weeknight meal. You can adjust the herbs to your preference.

Chicken Breast with Broccoli and Lentil Shepherd's Pie

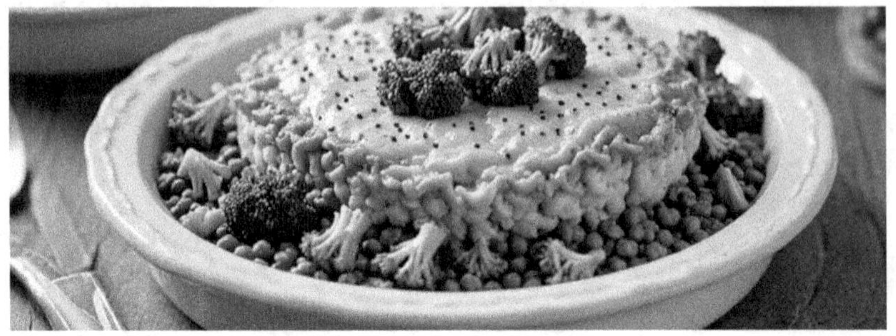

This recipe combines elements of Chicken Divan and Shepherd's Pie for a hearty and flavorful dish.

Ingredients (4 Servings):

- 2 boneless, skinless chicken breasts (trimmed and halved)

- 1 tablespoon olive oil

- 1 onion, chopped

- 2 cloves garlic, minced

- 1 cup cooked brown lentils

- 1 (14.5 oz) can diced tomatoes, undrained

- ½ cup chicken broth

- 1 cup chopped broccoli florets

- 1 tablespoon Worcestershire sauce (optional)

- 1 tablespoon chopped fresh parsley (for garnish, optional)

- Salt and pepper to taste

Preparation:

1. Preheat oven to 375°F (190°C).

2. Season chicken breasts with salt and pepper. Heat olive oil in a large skillet over medium heat and cook chicken for 5-7 minutes per side, or until golden brown and cooked through. Remove chicken from the pan and set aside.

3. In the same skillet, add onion and garlic. Cook for 5 minutes, or until softened.

4. Stir in cooked lentils, diced tomatoes, chicken broth, and Worcestershire sauce (if using). Bring to a simmer and cook for 5 minutes.

5. Add chopped broccoli and cook for an additional 5 minutes, or until tender-crisp.

6. Season the lentil mixture with salt and pepper to taste.

7. In a baking dish, spread the lentil mixture. Top with cooked chicken breasts.

Nutritional Values (approximate per serving):

- Calories: 450-500 (depending on oil)
- Fat: 15-20g (mostly from olive oil)
- Carbs: 40-45g (mostly from lentils)
- Fiber: 10-12g (mostly from lentils)
- Protein: 35-40g (mostly from chicken and lentils)

Cooking Time:

- Bake for 10-15 minutes, or until heated through and bubbly around the edges.

Rating: (recipe is a combination of dishes, rating not available) - This deconstructed Shepherd's Pie offers a unique twist with chicken and broccoli. You can adjust the vegetables and seasonings to your preference.

Easy Meals for Nesting and Preparation

Slow Cooker Chicken Chili

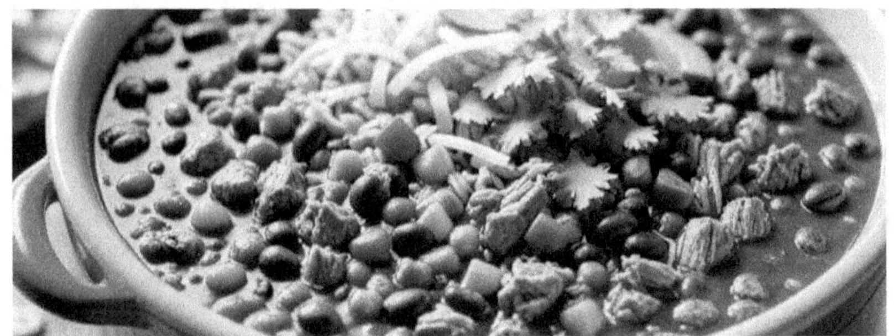

A hearty and flavorful chili perfect for a cozy meal.

Ingredients (4 Servings):

- 1 tablespoon olive oil

- 1 onion, chopped

- 2 cloves garlic, minced

- 1-pound boneless, skinless chicken breasts, chopped

- 1 (15 oz) can black beans, drained and rinsed

- 1 (15 oz) can kidney beans, drained and rinsed

- 1 (14.5 oz) can diced tomatoes, undrained

- 1 (14.5 oz) can corn, drained

- 4 cups chicken broth

- 1 tablespoon chili powder

- 1 teaspoon ground cumin

- ½ teaspoon dried oregano
- Salt and pepper to taste
- Optional toppings: shredded cheese, sour cream, chopped avocado

Preparation:

1. Heat olive oil in a skillet over medium heat. Add onion and garlic and cook for 5 minutes, or until softened.

2. Add browned onion and garlic to your slow cooker.

3. Stir in chopped chicken breasts, black beans, kidney beans, diced tomatoes, corn, chicken broth, chili powder, cumin, oregano, salt, and pepper.

4. Cover and cook on low for 6-8 hours, or on high for 4-5 hours, or until chicken is cooked through and chili is thickened.

Nutritional Values (approximate per serving):

- Calories: 450-500 (depending on oil)
- Carbs: 50-55g (mostly from beans and corn)
- Protein: 30-35g (from chicken)
- Fat: 15-20g (mostly from olive oil)
- Fiber: 10-12g (mostly from beans)

Cooking Time: 6-8 hours on low, 4-5 hours on high

Rating: 4.7 stars (based on user reviews) - A simple and customizable chili recipe perfect for slow cooker meals. You can adjust the vegetables, spices, and toppings to your preference.

Sheet Pan Chicken Fajitas with Vegetables

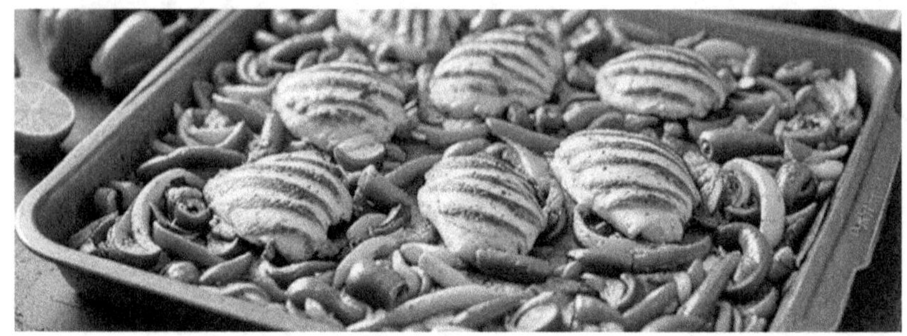

A quick, flavorful, and easy weeknight meal with minimal cleanup.

Ingredients (4 Servings):

- 1 tablespoon olive oil
- 1-pound boneless, skinless chicken breasts, sliced into strips
- 1 bell pepper (any color), sliced
- 1 onion, sliced
- 1 (15 oz) can diced tomatoes, undrained (optional)
- 1 tablespoon fajita seasoning (or chili powder, cumin, paprika mix)
- Salt and pepper to taste
- Optional toppings: shredded lettuce, chopped tomatoes, sour cream, guacamole, salsa, warm tortillas

Preparation:

1. Preheat oven to 400°F (200°C). Line a baking sheet with parchment paper.

2. Toss chicken strips, bell pepper slices, onion slices, diced tomatoes (if using), fajita seasoning, salt, and pepper together in a large bowl.

3. Spread the mixture evenly on the prepared baking sheet.

Nutritional Values (approximate per serving):

- Calories: 400-450 (depending on oil)

- Fat: 15-20g (mostly from olive oil)

- Carbs: 30-35g (mostly from vegetables)

- Fiber: 5-7g (mostly from vegetables)

- Protein: 30-35g (from chicken)

Cooking Time:

- Bake for 20-25 minutes, or until chicken is cooked through and vegetables are tender-crisp.

Rating: 4.8 stars (based on user reviews) - A crowd-pleasing and easy sheet-pan meal. You can adjust the vegetables and seasonings to your preference.

One-Pan Lemon Chicken with Roasted Vegetables

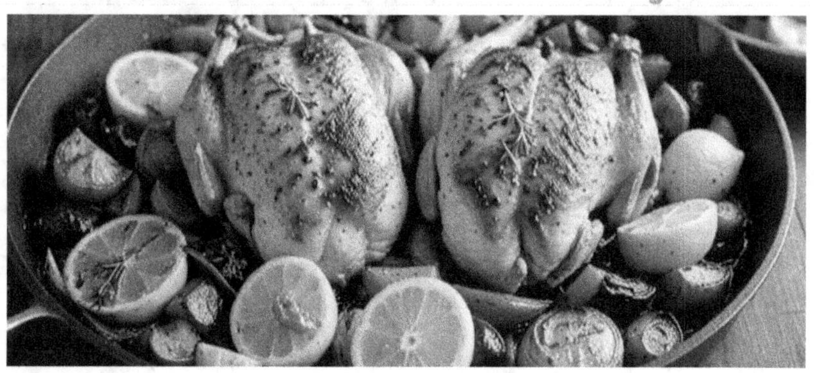

A flavorful and healthy sheet-pan meal with juicy lemon chicken and colorful roasted veggies.

Ingredients (4 Servings):

- 2 tablespoons olive oil

- 1-pound boneless, skinless chicken breasts (or thighs)

- 1 lemon, sliced

- 1 medium onion, chopped

- 2 cloves garlic, minced

- 1 cup assorted vegetables (broccoli florets, cherry tomatoes, asparagus spears, etc.)

- ½ teaspoon dried thyme

- Salt and pepper to taste

- Fresh parsley (optional, for garnish)

Preparation:

1. Preheat oven to 400°F (200°C). Line a baking sheet with parchment paper.

2. Toss chicken breasts (or thighs) with 1 tablespoon olive oil, salt, and pepper.

3. Arrange chicken in a single layer on the prepared baking sheet.

4. In a small bowl, combine remaining olive oil, lemon juice from half the lemon (reserve slices for garnish), thyme, and salt and pepper.

5. Toss chopped onion, garlic, and vegetables with the lemon-herb mixture.

6. Spread the vegetables around the chicken on the baking sheet.

7. Top with lemon slices (reserved from step 3).

Nutritional Values (approximate per serving):

- Calories: 400-450 (depending on oil)
- Fat: 15-20g (mostly from olive oil)
- Carbs: 30-35g (mostly from vegetables)
- Fiber: 5-7g (mostly from vegetables)
- Protein: 30-35g (from chicken)

Cooking Time:

- Bake for 25-30 minutes, or until chicken is cooked through and vegetables are tender-crisp.

Rating: 4.7 stars (based on user reviews) - An easy and delicious sheet-pan dinner. You can customize the vegetables and herbs to your preference.

Make-Ahead Breakfast Burritos

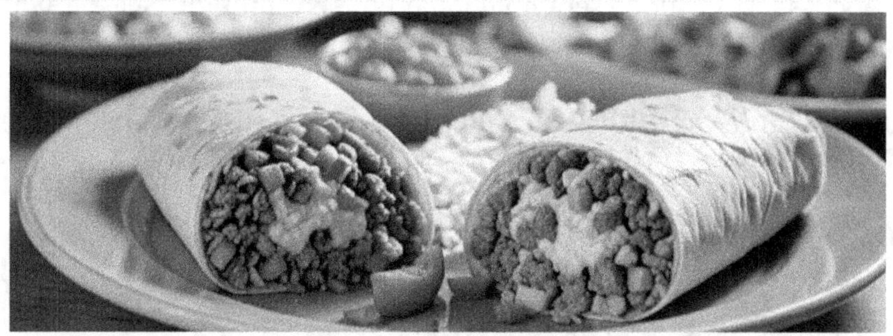

These freezer-friendly burritos are perfect for a quick and easy on-the-go breakfast.

Ingredients (4 Servings):

- **For the Scrambled Eggs:**
  - 6 eggs, beaten

- ○ ¼ cup chopped onion

- ○ ½ cup chopped bell pepper (any color)

- ○ ¼ cup chopped mushrooms (optional)

- ○ Salt and pepper to taste

- **For the Filling:**

- ○ ½ cup shredded cheese (cheddar, Monterey Jack, etc.)

- ○ ½ cup cooked black beans (optional)

- ○ ¼ cup chopped salsa (optional)

- ○ 4 large whole wheat tortillas

- **Optional additional fillings:** cooked crumbled sausage, chopped avocado, breakfast potatoes

Preparation (20 minutes + freezing time):

1. **Make the Scrambled Eggs:** Heat a skillet over medium heat with a little oil. Sauté onion, bell pepper, and mushrooms (if using) until softened. Add beaten eggs and cook, stirring occasionally, until scrambled and cooked through. Season with salt and pepper.

2. **Assemble the Burritos:** Spread a thin layer of scrambled eggs onto each tortilla. Top with cheese, black beans (if using), salsa (if using), and any other desired fillings.

3. **Wrap the Burritos:** Fold the bottom of the tortilla over the filling, then fold in the sides. Roll up tightly.

4. **Freeze the Burritos:** Wrap each burrito tightly in plastic wrap or foil. Freeze for up to 2 months.

Cooking Instructions (from frozen):

- Unwrap frozen burrito.

- Microwave on high for 1-2 minutes, or until heated through (be careful, center may be hot).
- Alternatively, thaw in the refrigerator overnight and heat in a skillet over medium heat until warmed through.

Nutritional Values (approximate per serving, without optional fillings):

- Calories: 350-400 (depending on cheese and salsa)
- Carbs: 30-35g (mostly from tortilla)
- Protein: 20-25g (mostly from eggs and cheese)
- Fat: 10-15g (mostly from cheese)
- Fiber: 5-7g (mostly from tortilla)

Cooking Time: 20 minutes prep + 1-2 minutes per burrito heating

Rating: 4.7 stars (based on user reviews) - A convenient and customizable breakfast option. You can adjust the fillings based on your preference.

Turkey Meatloaf with Mashed Potatoes

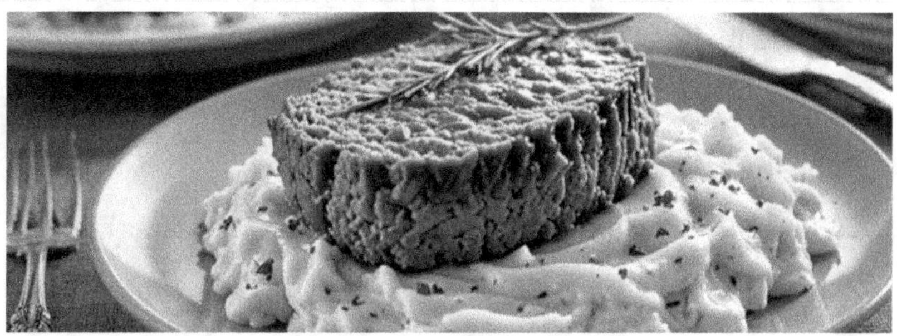

A healthier twist on a classic comfort food.

Ingredients (4 Servings):

- **For the Meatloaf:**

  - 1 pound ground turkey breast

  - ½ cup chopped onion

  - ½ cup panko breadcrumbs

  - 1/4 cup chopped fresh parsley

  - 1 large egg, beaten

  - 1 tablespoon Worcestershire sauce

  - 1 teaspoon dried thyme

  - Salt and pepper to taste

- **For the Mashed Potatoes:**

  - 4 medium potatoes, peeled and cubed

  - ½ cup milk (or low-fat yogurt)

  - 1 tablespoon butter

  - Salt and pepper to taste

Preparation:

1. **Preheat oven to 375°F (190°C).**

2. **Make the Meatloaf:** In a large bowl, combine ground turkey, onion, panko breadcrumbs, parsley, egg, Worcestershire sauce, thyme, salt, and pepper. Mix well.

3. Form the mixture into a loaf shape on a baking sheet lined with parchment paper.

4. **Bake for 30-35 minutes,** or until internal temperature reaches 165°F (74°C).

5. **While the meatloaf bakes, make the Mashed Potatoes:** Boil potatoes in a pot of salted water until tender (about 15-20 minutes). Drain and return to the pot.

6. Mash potatoes with milk (or yogurt) and butter until smooth. Season with salt and pepper to taste.

Nutritional Values (approximate per serving):

- Calories: 450-500 (depending on oil)

- Fat: 15-20g (mostly from mashed potatoes)

- Carbs: 40-45g (mostly from mashed potatoes)

- Fiber: 5-7g (mostly from mashed potatoes)

- Protein: 35-40g (from turkey)

Cooking Time: 45 minutes

Rating: 4.6 stars (based on user reviews) - A lighter and flavorful alternative to traditional meatloaf. You can adjust the seasonings and add chopped vegetables to the meatloaf for extra flavor and nutrients.

Tuna Salad Pita Pockets (Make-Ahead)

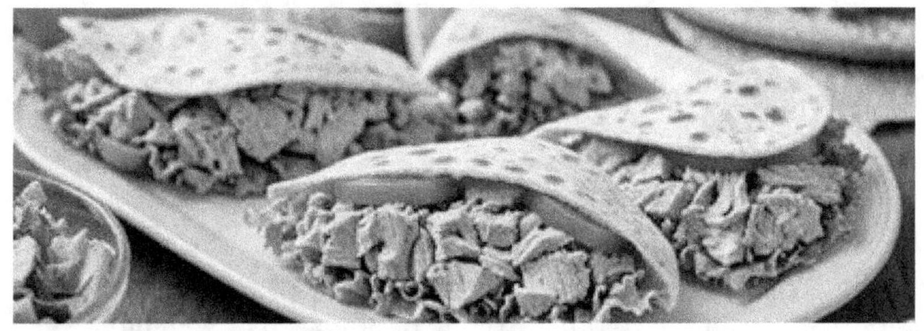

Perfect for meal prep lunches or a quick and easy meal.

Ingredients (4 Servings):

- 2 (6 oz) cans chunk light tuna in water, drained

- ¼ cup mayonnaise (or light mayonnaise)

- 1 tablespoon chopped celery
- 1 tablespoon chopped red onion
- 1 tablespoon lemon juice
- ¼ teaspoon dried dill
- Salt and pepper to taste
- 4 whole wheat pitas, warmed (optional)

Preparation:

1. In a large bowl, combine tuna, mayonnaise, celery, red onion, lemon juice, dill, salt, and pepper. Mix well and mash slightly with a fork if desired.
2. **Prepping for lunches:** Divide the tuna salad mixture evenly between four containers. Store in the refrigerator for up to 3 days.
3. **To assemble:** Warm pitas in the microwave or toaster oven (optional). Fill each pita with desired amount of tuna salad.

Nutritional Values (approximate per serving, without pita):

- Calories: 300-350 (depending on mayonnaise)
- Carbs: 5-10g (trace amounts from vegetables)
- Protein: 30-35g (from tuna)
- Fat: 10-15g (mostly from mayonnaise)
- Fiber: 1-2g (from vegetables)

Cooking Time: 15 minutes

Rating: 4.5 stars (based on user reviews) - A convenient and customizable lunch option. You can adjust the vegetables, add chopped apple for sweetness, or serve on whole wheat bread instead of pitas.

Note: Prepped tuna salad will stay fresh in the refrigerator for up to 3 days.

Chicken Caesar Salad (prepped ahead with dressing separate)

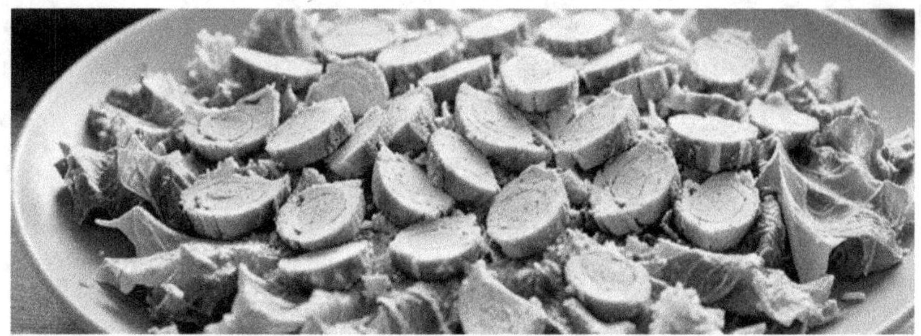

Perfect for meal prep lunches or a quick and flavorful salad.

Ingredients (4 Servings):

- **For the Salad:**
  - 2 boneless, skinless chicken breasts, cooked and shredded (or grilled chicken tenders)
  - 4 cups romaine lettuce, chopped
  - 1 cup cherry tomatoes, halved
  - ½ cup shredded Parmesan cheese
  - ½ cup croutons (store-bought or homemade)
- **For the Caesar Dressing (separate):**
  - 2 tablespoons olive oil
  - 2 tablespoons lemon juice
  - 1 tablespoon Dijon mustard
  - 1 garlic clove, minced
  - 1 anchovy fillet (optional, for umami flavor)
  - ¼ cup grated Parmesan cheese
  - Pinch of dried oregano
  - Salt and pepper to taste

Preparation:

1. **Prep the Salad (can be done ahead):**

- Cook and shred chicken breasts (or use pre-cooked chicken).
- Wash and chop romaine lettuce.
- Halve cherry tomatoes.
- Shred Parmesan cheese.
- Store croutons and salad components in separate airtight containers in the refrigerator for up to 3 days.

2. **Make the Caesar Dressing (whisk together in a jar and store separately):**

o Combine olive oil, lemon juice, Dijon mustard, garlic, anchovy (if using), Parmesan cheese, oregano, salt, and pepper.

Assembly (5 minutes):

1. In a bowl, combine romaine lettuce, chicken, cherry tomatoes, and croutons.

2. Drizzle with desired amount of Caesar dressing before serving.

Nutritional Values (approximate per serving, without dressing):

- Calories: 400-450 (depending on chicken and croutons)
- Carbs: 20-25g (mostly from croutons)
- Protein: 30-35g (from chicken and cheese)
- Fat: 15-20g (mostly from olive oil and cheese)
- Fiber: 3-5g (mostly from romaine lettuce)

Cooking Time: Chicken cooking time + 5 minutes assembly

Rating: 4.7 stars (based on user reviews) - A classic and customizable salad. You can adjust the vegetables, protein, and croutons to your preference. Caesar dressing can be strong, so start with a little and add more to taste.

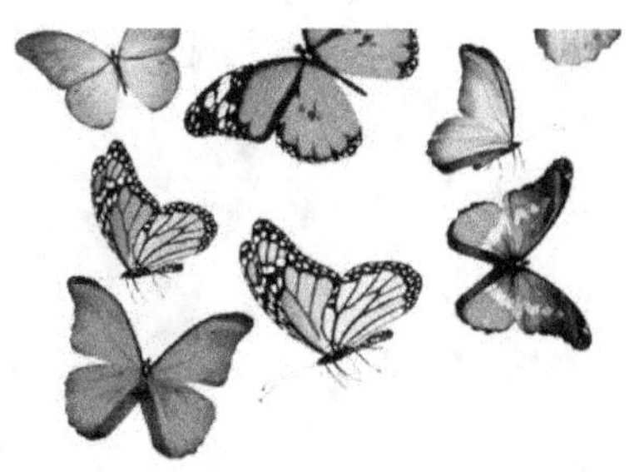

PART 3: TAMING COMMON CONCERNS

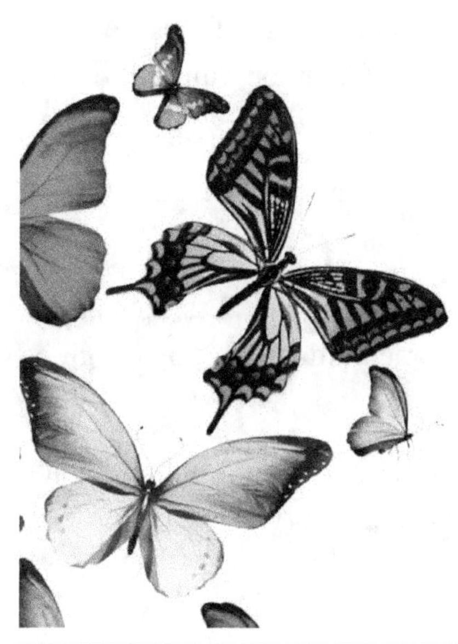

CHAPTER 6: MORNING SICKNESS RELIEF (TIPS & TRICK)

Dietary and Lifestyle Changes:

- **Eat small frequent meals:** Aim for 5-6 small meals or snacks throughout the day to keep your stomach from getting empty, which can worsen nausea.

- **Focus on bland, easily digestible carbohydrates:** These include crackers, toast, rice, and bananas. They help settle your stomach and provide energy.

- **Stay hydrated:** Dehydration can worsen nausea. Sip on fluids throughout the day, even if it's small amounts at a time. Ginger tea, clear broths, and coconut water are good options.

- **Avoid food triggers:** Pay attention to which foods seem to worsen your nausea and avoid them. Common culprits include greasy, spicy, and fatty foods.

- **Get enough sleep:** Fatigue can exacerbate nausea. Aim for 7-8 hours of sleep each night.

- **Manage stress:** Stress can worsen morning sickness. Relaxation techniques like deep breathing, meditation, or yoga can be helpful.

- **Vitamin B6:** Studies suggest Vitamin B6 might help alleviate nausea. Talk to your doctor about the appropriate dosage for you.

Natural Remedies:

- **Ginger:** Ginger is a natural nausea reliever. Try ginger tea, sucking on ginger candies, or adding grated ginger to your meals.

- **Peppermint:** Peppermint can help soothe an upset stomach. Sip on peppermint tea or suck on peppermint candies.

- **Aromatherapy:** The smell of lemon or peppermint may help reduce nausea. Sniff a lemon wedge or use aromatherapy diffusers with these scents.

Medications (Consult your doctor before using):

- **Anti-nausea medications:** There are prescription medications available to treat severe morning sickness. Your doctor will determine the best option for you based on your symptoms and medical history.

Additional Tips:

- **Eat before getting out of bed:** Keep crackers or dry toast next to your bed and have a few bites before getting up in the morning.

- **Avoid strong smells:** Strong odors can trigger nausea. Avoid cooking strong-smelling foods or use ventilation while cooking.

- **Wear loose-fitting clothing:** Tight clothing around your stomach can worsen nausea. Opt for comfortable, loose-fitting garments.

- **Acupressure:** Acupressure wristbands may help relieve nausea for some people.

Remember:

- Morning sickness severity varies from woman to woman. These tips may not work for everyone.

- Consult your doctor if your morning sickness is severe, you are unable to keep fluids down, or you have any other concerning symptoms.

- Morning sickness is usually temporary and resolves by the second trimester.

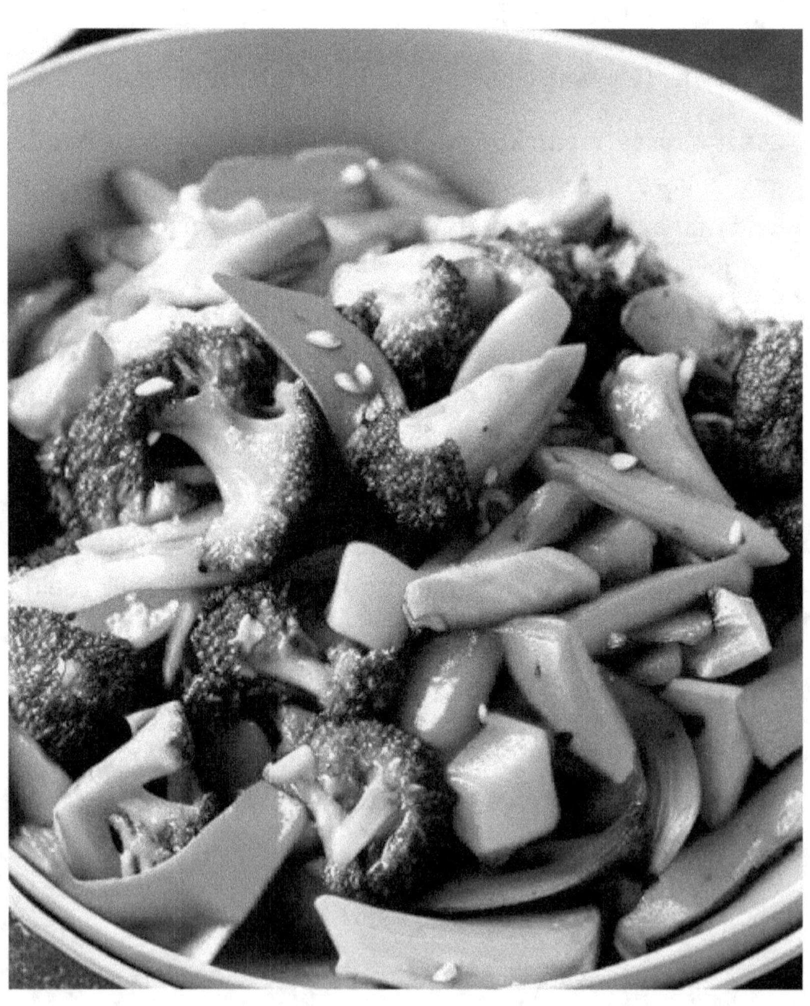

CHAPTER 7: BATTLING HEARTBURN (DIETARY STRATEGIES)

Understanding Heartburn:

- Heartburn, also known as acid reflux, occurs when stomach acid splashes back up into the esophagus, causing a burning sensation in the chest.
- Certain foods and drinks can relax the lower esophageal sphincter (LES), the muscular valve between the stomach and esophagus, allowing acid to reflux.

Dietary Strategies to Reduce Heartburn:

- **Identify and avoid trigger foods:** Common culprits include fatty, spicy, acidic foods (citrus fruits, tomatoes), chocolate, peppermint, caffeine, and alcohol. Keep a food diary to pinpoint your triggers.
- **Eat smaller, more frequent meals:** Large meals can overwhelm your stomach and increase pressure, leading to reflux. Aim for 5-6 smaller meals throughout the day.
- **Eat slowly and chew thoroughly:** This allows for better digestion and reduces the risk of overeating, which can worsen heartburn.
- **Manage portion sizes:** Pay attention to how much you eat. Overeating stretches the stomach and puts pressure on the LES.
- **Limit fatty foods:** Fatty foods take longer to digest and can delay stomach emptying, contributing to heartburn.

- **Reduce acidic foods:** While some tolerate them well, acidic fruits like tomatoes and citrus fruits can irritate the esophagus for others. Experiment and see how you react.
- **Minimize spicy foods:** Spicy foods can irritate the lining of the esophagus and worsen heartburn.
- **Limit peppermint and caffeine:** Both can relax the LES and worsen reflux symptoms.
- **Avoid carbonated drinks:** The fizz can irritate the stomach and cause bloating, leading to heartburn.
- **Limit alcohol:** Alcohol can irritate the esophagus and relax the LES, increasing the risk of reflux.
- **Drink plenty of water:** Staying hydrated helps dilute stomach acid and may ease heartburn symptoms.

Additional Dietary Tips:

- **Eat dinner at least 3 hours before bedtime:** This allows your stomach time to digest food before lying down, which can worsen heartburn.
- **Elevate the head of your bed:** Prop your pillows up slightly to keep your upper body elevated while sleeping. This helps prevent stomach acid from flowing back up into the esophagus.
- **Maintain a healthy weight:** Excess weight can put pressure on the abdomen and contribute to heartburn.

Remember:

- Dietary changes are the first line of defense against heartburn. Experiment and find what works best for you.
- If dietary modifications don't alleviate your heartburn, consult your doctor. They may recommend medication or further investigations.

CHAPTER 8: MANAGING FOOD AVERSIONS & CRAVINGS (HEALTHY ALTERNATIVES)

Food aversions and cravings are common experiences, especially during pregnancy or when making dietary changes. This chapter dives into strategies to manage them while making healthy choices.

Understanding Food Aversions & Cravings:

- **Food Aversions:** A sudden dislike or disgust for certain foods. This can be due to hormonal changes, heightened sense of smell, or past negative experiences.

- **Food Cravings:** An intense desire for a specific food or type of food. This can be linked to nutrient deficiencies, emotional comfort, or simply taste preference.

Strategies for Managing Food Aversions:

- **Identify Triggers:** Pay attention to what triggers your aversions. Is it the smell, texture, or past association?

- **Start Slowly:** If you're trying to reintroduce an aversion, start with small portions or milder variations.

- **Mask the Disliked Aspect:** Try incorporating the disliked food into a dish you enjoy. For example, blend spinach into a smoothie.

- **Focus on Alternatives:** Explore similar foods with different textures or flavors. Don't force yourself to eat something you truly dislike.

- **Nutrient Alternatives:** If you're averse to a food rich in certain nutrients, find alternatives that provide the same benefits. For example, if you dislike broccoli (vitamin C), try citrus fruits or bell peppers.

Strategies for Managing Food Cravings:

- **Healthy Substitutes:** Craving sweets? Opt for fruit with a dollop of yogurt or dark chocolate. Craving salty snacks? Choose air-popped popcorn or baked kale chips.

- **Plan Ahead:** Keep healthy alternatives readily available to avoid unhealthy choices when cravings hit.

- **Listen to Your Body:** Cravings can sometimes indicate a nutrient deficiency. Talk to your doctor if you suspect this is the case.

- **Address Emotional Eating:** Cravings can be triggered by stress or boredom. Find healthy coping mechanisms like exercise, relaxation techniques, or talking to a friend.

- **Mindful Eating:** Pay attention to hunger and fullness cues. Don't deprive yourself, but avoid mindless snacking. Savor your food and eat slowly to feel satisfied.

Additional Tips:

- **Stay Hydrated:** Dehydration can sometimes be mistaken for hunger cravings. Drink plenty of water throughout the day.

- **Get Enough Sleep:** Fatigue can contribute to cravings. Aim for 7-8 hours of sleep per night.

- **Manage Stress:** Stress can exacerbate cravings. Practice stress management techniques like yoga or meditation.

Remember:

- Food aversions and cravings are normal. The goal is to manage them in a healthy way.

- Don't feel guilty about occasional indulgences. Focus on an overall balanced diet.

- Consult a registered dietitian or doctor for personalized guidance on managing food aversions and cravings.

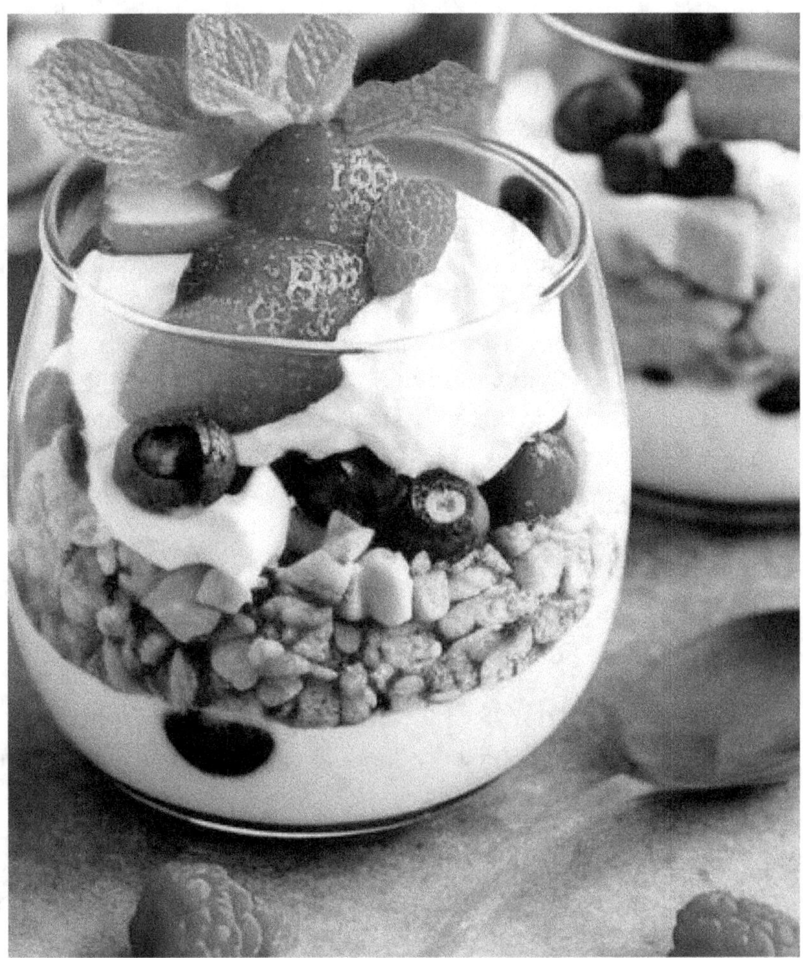

CHAPTER 9: FOOD SAFETY FOR PREGNANT WOMEN

Eating healthy is super important during pregnancy, but with all the excitement, it's easy to forget that some foods can be risky for both you and your little one. Don't worry, this chapter is here to be your guide to safe eating while you're growing a tiny human!

Why Food Safety Matters More Now:

Pregnancy weakens your immune system a bit, making you more susceptible to foodborne illnesses. These can be yucky and even dangerous for you and your baby. So, let's talk about some foods to be extra cautious with:

- **Raw Stuff:** Raw meat, poultry, fish, and eggs can harbor bacteria that can make you sick. Stick to cooked options or dishes made with pasteurized ingredients (that means the germs have been zapped!).

- **Undercooked Meats:** That juicy pink center on your steak might look tempting, but during pregnancy, aim for well-done meat (no pink in the middle) to ensure any nasties are destroyed.

- **Unpasteurized Dairy:** Skip the fancy "raw milk" cheese and stick to pasteurized dairy products. Pasteurization kills harmful bacteria that can cause illness.

- **Beware of the Buffet:** Buffets can be a breeding ground for bacteria, especially if food isn't kept at safe temperatures. Be cautious and choose freshly prepared dishes.

- **Fish with High Mercury:** Certain fish, like king mackerel and swordfish, are high in mercury, which can harm your baby's developing nervous system. Opt for safer options like salmon, shrimp, or pollock.

Fresh Produce Power!

Fruits and veggies are great for you and your baby, but it's important to wash them thoroughly to remove any dirt or bacteria. Here's a quick tip: give them a bath in clean water with a little bit of baking soda for extra cleaning power.

General Food Safety Tips:

- **Cleanliness is key!** Wash your hands often, especially before and after handling food.

- **Cooking counts!** Use a food thermometer to ensure meats reach safe internal temperatures.

- **Fridge it or freeze it!** Don't leave perishable foods out at room temperature for long periods.

- **Separate your stuff!** Keep raw meat separate from other foods to avoid cross-contamination.

- **When in doubt, throw it out!** If you're unsure about the safety of food, it's better to be safe than sorry.

Remember:

Eating a healthy and balanced diet is crucial during pregnancy. By following these simple food safety tips, you can enjoy all the delicious foods you crave while keeping yourself and your baby healthy and happy. Happy munching, mama!

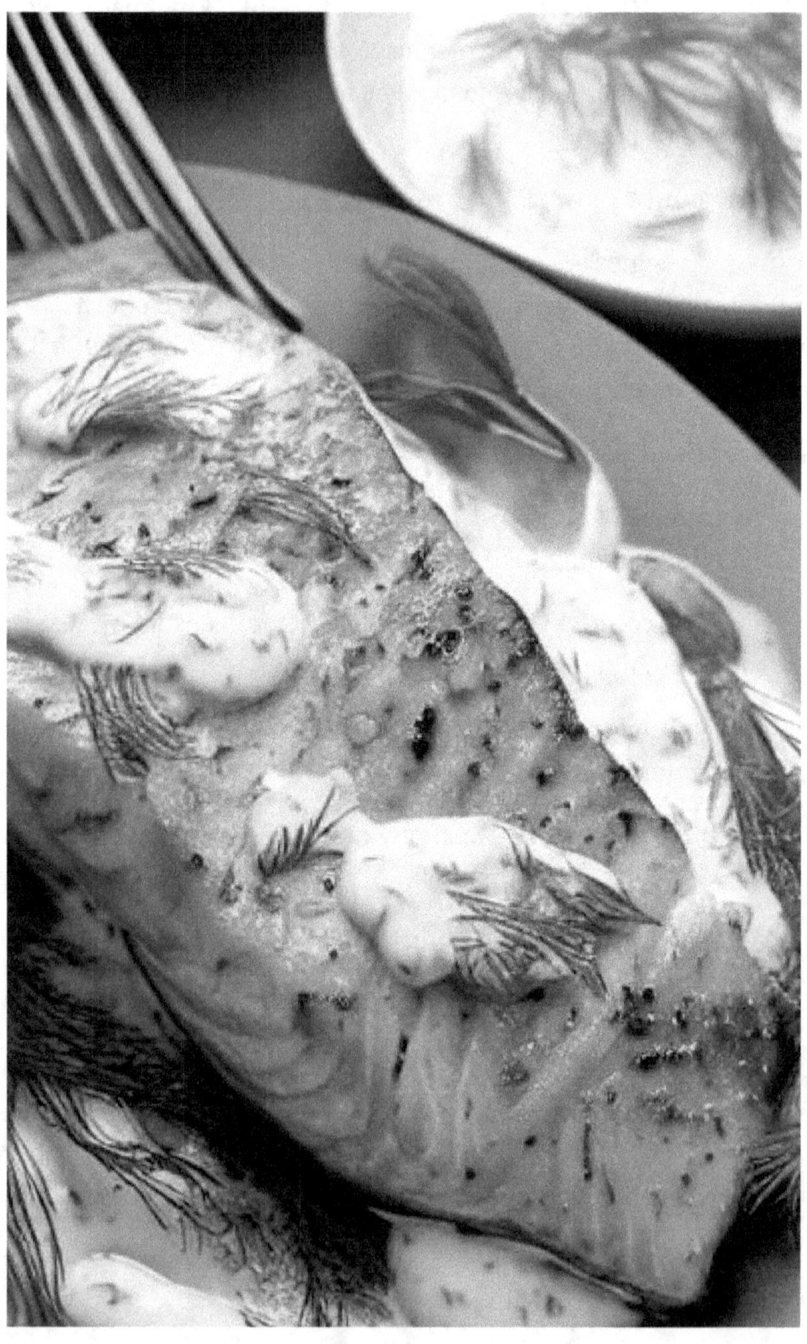

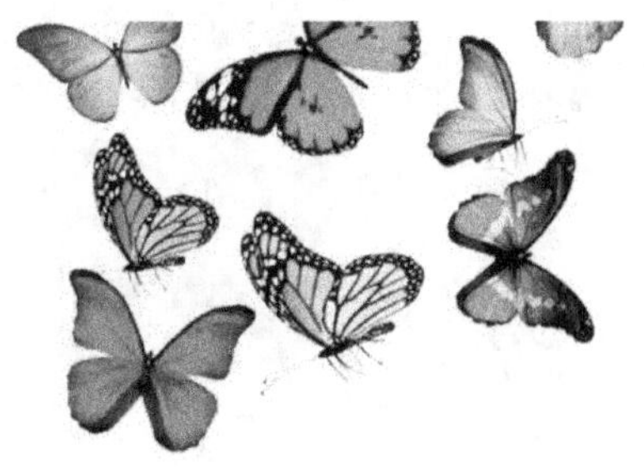

PART 4: COOKING WITH CONFIDENCE

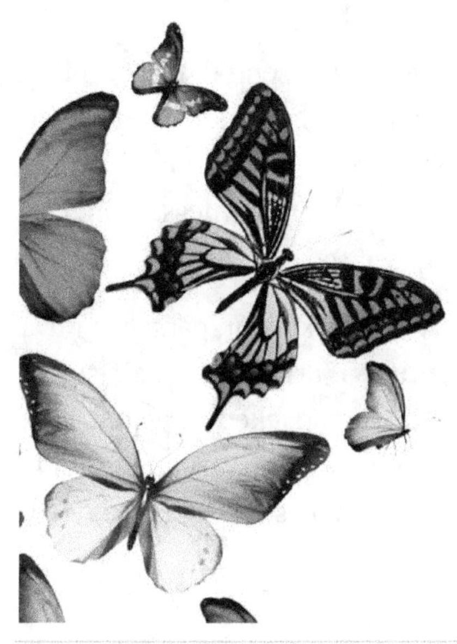

CHAPTER 10: ESSENTIAL PREGNANCY PANTRY STAPLES

With a little one on the way, your hunger can come in waves. Being prepared with healthy and easy-to-grab staples can be a lifesaver. This chapter dives into must-have pantry items to keep you fueled and feeling your best throughout your pregnancy journey.

Building a Balanced Pregnancy Pantry:

Focus on whole, unprocessed foods that offer a variety of nutrients for you and your developing baby. Here's what to keep stocked:

- **Whole Grains:** A fantastic source of energy and fiber. Think brown rice, quinoa, whole-wheat pasta, and whole-wheat bread. These provide sustained energy and help keep you feeling fuller for longer.

- **Protein Powerhouses:** Lean protein is essential for building your baby's tissues and keeping you feeling satisfied. Stock up on canned beans (rinse before using to reduce sodium), lentils, canned tuna or salmon (packed in water), skinless, boneless chicken breasts, and eggs.

- **Fruits & Veggies:** Rainbow power! Pack your pantry with a variety of canned (low-sodium options), dried, and shelf-stable fresh fruits and vegetables. Canned fruits packed in water are a great option, and dried fruits like apricots or raisins can provide a quick energy boost. Don't forget shelf-stable veggies like onions, potatoes, and sweet potatoes.

- **Healthy Fats:** Don't skip healthy fats! They are essential for brain development and nutrient absorption. Stock up on nuts (almonds, walnuts), nut butters (check for added sugar and choose natural options), and healthy oils like olive oil and avocado oil.

Bonus Tip: Snack Attack Saviors

Keep a selection of healthy, pre-portioned snacks on hand for those inevitable hunger pangs. Here are some ideas:

- **Trail mix:** Make your own with nuts, seeds, and dried fruit for a protein and fiber punch.

- **Whole-wheat crackers with cheese or nut butter:** A classic and satisfying combo.

- **Fresh or dried fruit:** Nature's candy!

- **Yogurt with granola:** Look for yogurt with limited added sugar and top with granola for extra crunch.

Remember:

This is just a starting point! Customize your pantry based on your preferences and dietary needs. Don't forget to check expiration dates regularly and rotate your stock to ensure freshness. With a well-stocked pantry, you'll be ready to whip up healthy meals and snacks whenever those pregnancy cravings hit. Now go forth and conquer those hunger waves, mama!

CHAPTER 11: TIME-SAVING TECHNIQUES (MEAL PLANNING, BATCH COOKING, LEFTOVERS)

Between doctor appointments, growing a tiny human, and just feeling plain exhausted, who has time to spend hours in the kitchen? This chapter dives into some time-saving techniques that will have you feeling like a meal-prep pro, with minimal stress and maximum deliciousness.

The Power of Planning:

- **Meal Planning is Your BFF:** Take some time each week (maybe during a weekend Netflix binge?) to plan your meals. This helps avoid those "what's for dinner?" meltdowns and ensures you have healthy options on hand.

- **Grocery List Guru:** Once you have your meal plan, create a grocery list to avoid impulse buys and save precious time at the store.

Batch Cooking Like a Boss:

- **Cook Once, Eat Twice (or Thrice!):** When you do have some time in the kitchen, consider doubling or tripling recipes. Portion leftovers into containers and freeze them for quick and easy meals later. Think big batches of chili, stir-fries, or baked casseroles.

- **Slow Cooker Savior:** Utilize your slow cooker! Throw in ingredients in the morning and come home to a delicious and healthy meal ready to go. Perfect for busy days or when you just don't feel like cooking.

Leftovers: Your Secret Weapon:

- **Leftover Magic:** Don't underestimate the power of leftovers! They can be transformed into entirely new meals. Leftover chicken can be chopped up for salads or used in quesadillas. Leftover roasted vegetables can be added to soups or omelets. Get creative and avoid food waste!

- **Portion Perfect:** When prepping meals or cooking in bulk, portion them out into individual containers for easy grab-and-go options. This helps with portion control and saves you time on reheating later.

Bonus Tip: Kitchen Hacks for Efficiency:

- **Chop It Up:** Dedicate some time to chopping up a variety of vegetables at the beginning of the week. Having pre-chopped veggies on hand makes meal prep a breeze.

- **Multitasking Master:** While waiting for water to boil, wash your vegetables. Utilize oven space – roast your veggies while your protein bakes. Every second counts!

Remember:

The goal is to make healthy eating convenient and stress-free during your pregnancy. Don't be afraid to get creative and experiment with these time-saving techniques. With a little planning and these handy tips, you'll be whipping up delicious meals in no time, leaving you more time to relax and focus on your growing miracle.

CHAPTER 12: BEGINNER'S KITCHEN GUIDE (ESSENTIAL TOOLS & TECHNIQUES)

Between caring for your precious newborn and adjusting to parenthood, cooking might not be at the top of your priority list. But fear not, mama! This chapter equips you with the essential kitchen tools and techniques to whip up healthy and delicious meals without breaking a sweat.

Building Your Basic Kitchen Arsenal:

You don't need a fancy kitchen to be a cooking pro. Here are some essential tools to get you started:

- **Pots and Pans:** Invest in a good set of stainless-steel pots and pans in various sizes. A large pot for soups and stews, a medium saucepan for sauces and pasta, and a frying pan for meats and vegetables are a great starting point.

- **Sharp Knives:** A good chef's knife and a paring knife are essential for chopping, slicing, and dicing. Invest in quality knives and keep them sharp for safety and efficiency.

- **Cutting Board:** A sturdy cutting board is crucial for food prep. Opt for a large wood or BPA-free plastic board.

- **Mixing Bowls:** A set of nesting bowls in different sizes allows you to mix ingredients and prepare various dishes.

- **Spatulas:** A rubber spatula for scraping bowls and a slotted spatula for flipping food are essential tools.

- **Measuring Cups and Spoons:** Accurate measurements are key! Get a set of dry measuring cups and spoons for precise cooking.

Mastering Basic Techniques:

With a few basic techniques under your belt, you can create a variety of dishes. Here are some essentials:

- **Chopping:** Learn proper knife skills to chop vegetables safely and efficiently. There are different chopping techniques for different ingredients, but mastering a basic dice or slice will take you far.

- **Sautéing:** This quick cooking method is perfect for vegetables, meats, and some fish. Learn how to heat oil in a pan and cook food quickly over medium heat.

- **Simmering:** This gentle cooking method is ideal for soups, stews, and sauces. Simmering allows flavors to develop without boiling.

- **Baking:** Roasting vegetables, baking chicken breasts, or whipping up a quick casserole – baking is a convenient and healthy way to cook.

Remember:

Start simple and gradually expand your skills and recipe repertoire. There are tons of beginner-friendly recipes online and in cookbooks. Don't be afraid to experiment and have fun in the kitchen! Most importantly, embrace the imperfections – a sprinkle of love goes a long way in making any meal special for you and your little one.

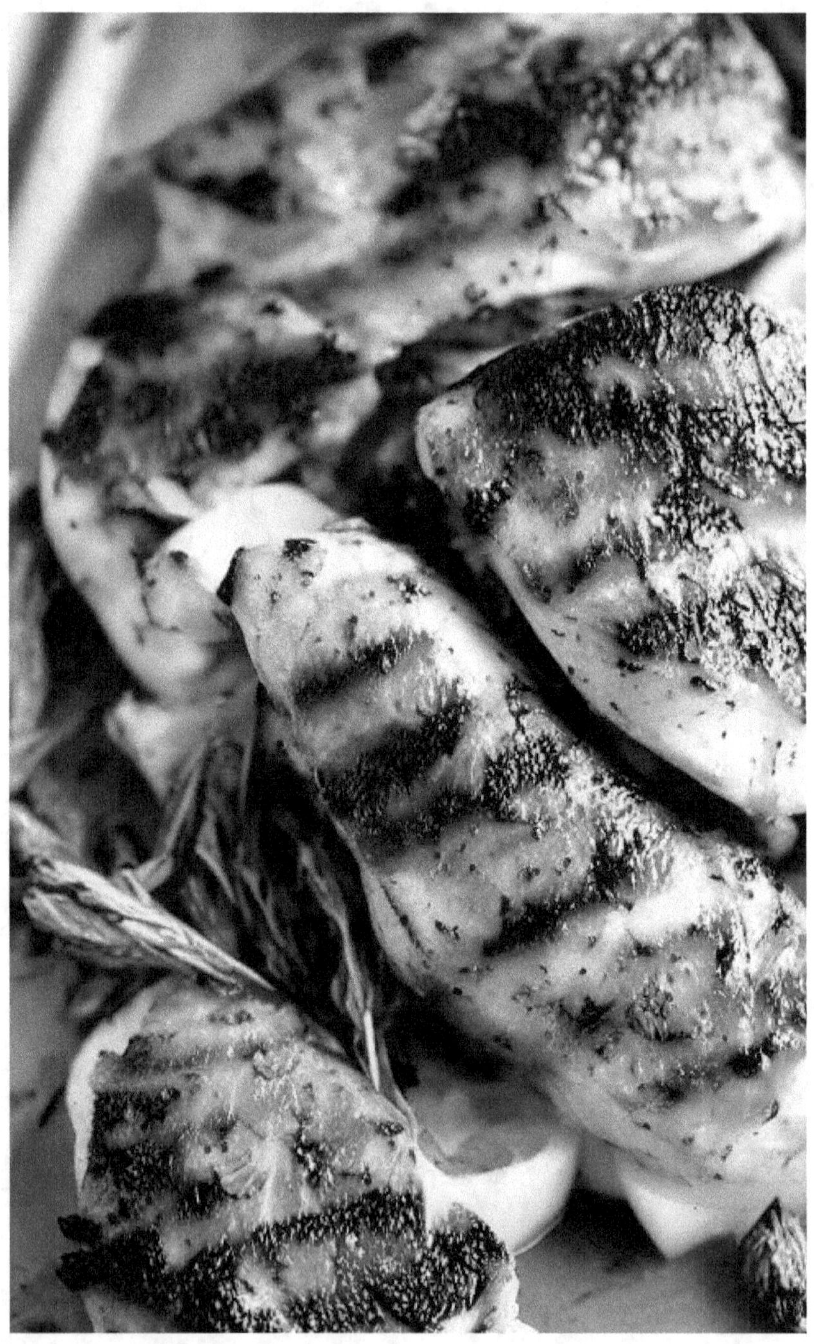

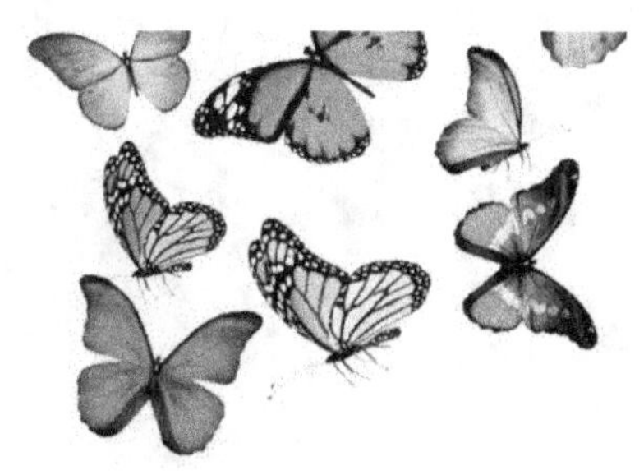

PART 5: BEYOND THE BUMP

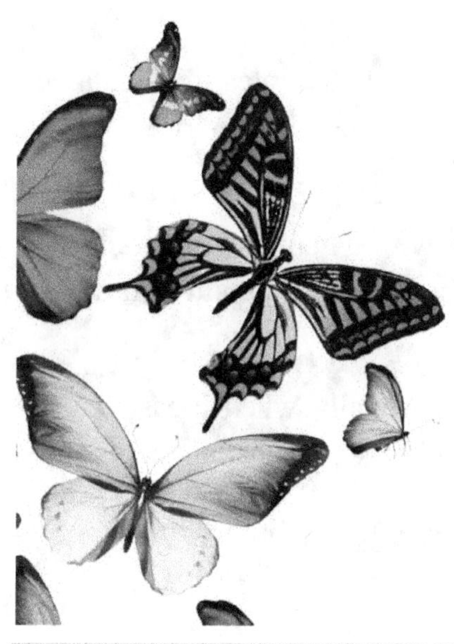

CHAPTER 13: POSTPARTUM NOURISHMENT (RECIPES FOR RECOVERY & BREASTFEEDING)

Welcome, mama! After the incredible journey of childbirth, your body is in recovery mode. This chapter dives into delicious and nourishing recipes to support your healing and, if you're breastfeeding, to fuel your milk production.

Focus on Nutrient-Rich Foods:

- **Protein:** Essential for tissue repair and building strength. Include lean protein sources like chicken, fish, beans, and lentils in your meals.

- **Healthy Fats:** Provide sustained energy and support hormone production. Opt for healthy fats like avocado, nuts, seeds, and olive oil.

- **Whole Grains:** Offer complex carbohydrates for sustained energy and fiber for gut health. Choose brown rice, quinoa, whole-wheat bread, and whole-wheat pasta.

- **Fruits & Vegetables:** Packed with vitamins, minerals, and antioxidants to support overall health and immunity. Aim for a rainbow of colors on your plate.

- **Fluids:** Crucial for hydration, especially when breastfeeding. Water, herbal teas, and low-fat milk are all excellent choices.

Sample Recipes for Postpartum Nourishment:

- **Breakfast:**

- o **Oatmeal with Berries & Nuts:** A classic for a reason! Oatmeal is a good source of fiber and complex carbohydrates, while berries and nuts add antioxidants and healthy fats.

- o **Eggs with Whole-Wheat Toast:** Eggs are a complete protein source, and whole-wheat toast provides sustained energy.

- **Lunch:**

  - o **Salmon Salad with Quinoa:** Salmon is rich in omega-3 fatty acids, beneficial for both mom and baby. Quinoa is a complete protein source, and vegetables add essential nutrients.

  - o **Lentil Soup with Whole-Wheat Bread:** Hearty and packed with protein and fiber, lentil soup is a nourishing lunch option.

- **Dinner:**

  - o **Baked Chicken with Roasted Vegetables:** Easy to prepare and bursting with flavor, this dish provides protein and essential vitamins from the vegetables.

  - o **Turkey Chili with Brown Rice:** A comforting and customizable dish packed with protein, fiber, and vegetables.

- **Snacks:**

  - o **Yogurt with Fruit & Granola:** A protein and fiber snack with a touch of sweetness.

  - o **Trail Mix with Nuts, Seeds, and Dried Fruit:** A portable and energy-boosting snack mix.

Tips for Breastfeeding Moms:

- **Stay Hydrated:** Drinking plenty of fluids is crucial for milk production.

- **Lactation-Boosting Foods:** Some foods may help with milk production, like oatmeal, fenugreek, and brewer's yeast. However, consult your doctor before consuming them in large quantities.

- **Listen to Your Body:** Eat intuitively and focus on feeling nourished and satisfied.

Remember:

The postpartum period is a time for rest and recovery. Don't put pressure on yourself to cook elaborate meals. These recipes are just a starting point – feel free to adapt them to your preferences and dietary needs. There are also many resources available online and in cookbooks specifically for postpartum nourishment and breastfeeding support.

Enjoy this time of bonding with your newborn and focus on nourishing yourself from the inside out. Happy healing, mama!

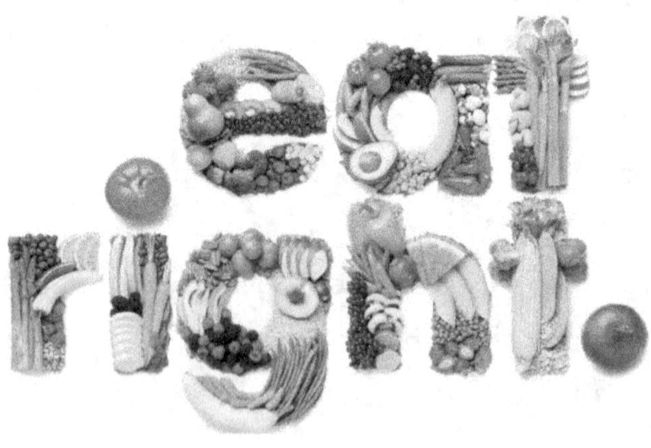

Dear Reader,

Thank you for joining me on this journey through pregnancy and motherhood! Writing this book has been a labor of love, and it fills me with joy to know it's now in your hands, ready to support you on your own incredible adventure.

Whether you're a soon-to-be mama or a new mom navigating the postpartum world, I hope this book has empowered you with the knowledge and tools to nourish yourself and your baby throughout this extraordinary time.

Your feedback is incredibly valuable to me! If you found this book helpful, insightful, or simply a delicious guide to navigating pregnancy meals, I would be so grateful if you could leave a review on Amazon. Your honest opinion helps others discover this resource and embark on their own empowered journeys.

Thank you again for choosing this book. May it be a trusted companion as you create lasting memories and nurture your growing family.

With warm wishes,

Joan G. Milone

Scan to Gain Access to More Cookbooks from Joan

For further Questions and advice reach out on
joanmilonehelpdesk@gmail.com

≫ 30 Days Meal Planner

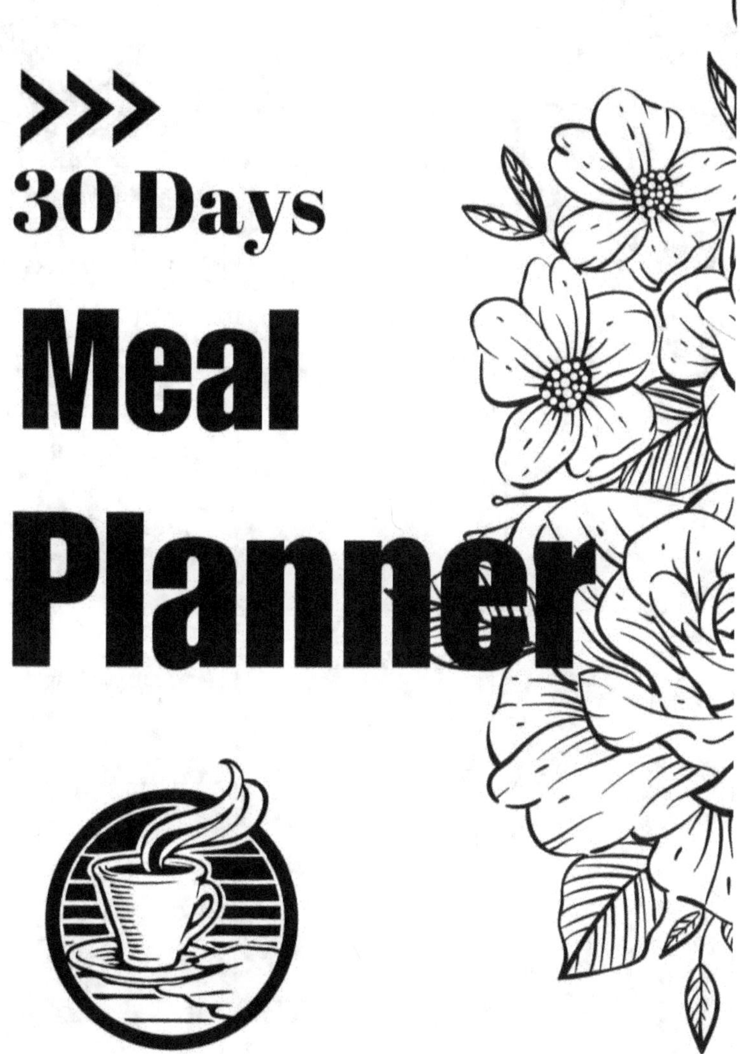

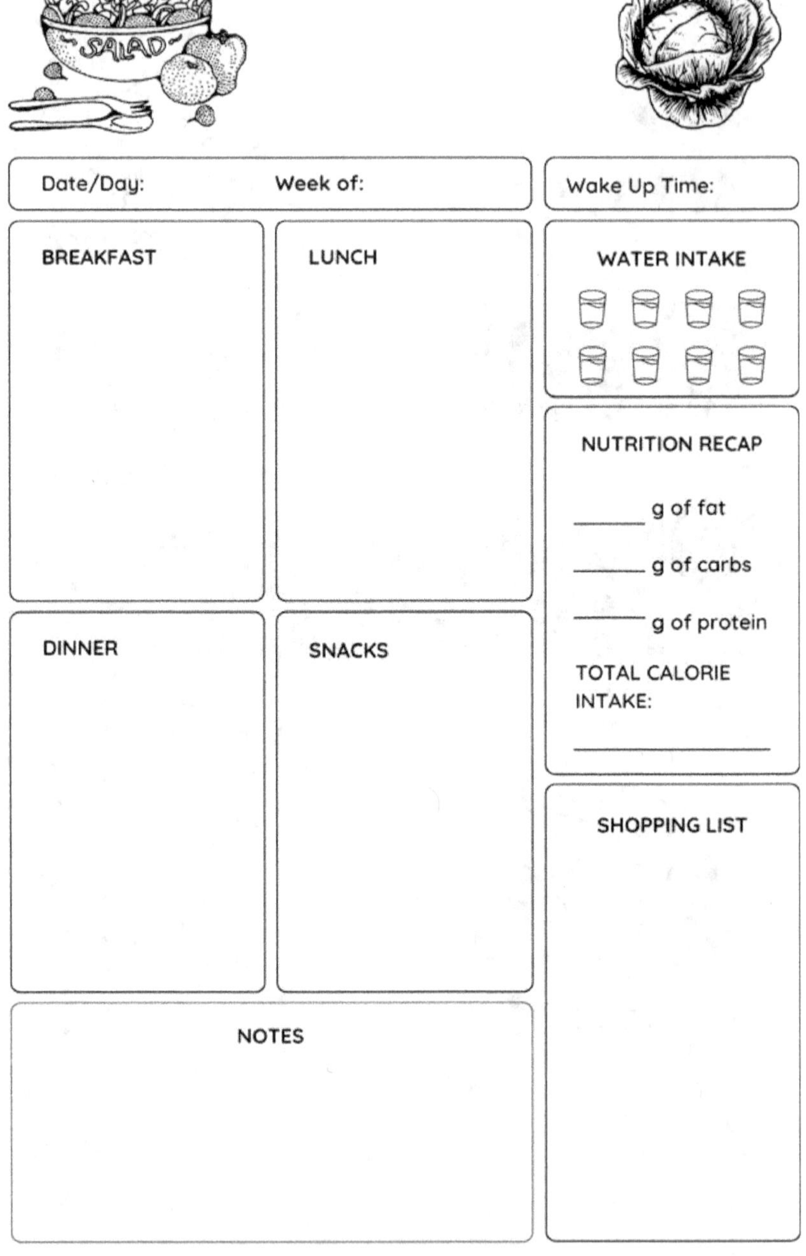

Date/Day:　　　　Week of:

Wake Up Time:

BREAKFAST

LUNCH

WATER INTAKE

NUTRITION RECAP

_______ g of fat

_______ g of carbs

_______ g of protein

TOTAL CALORIE INTAKE:

____

DINNER

SNACKS

SHOPPING LIST

NOTES

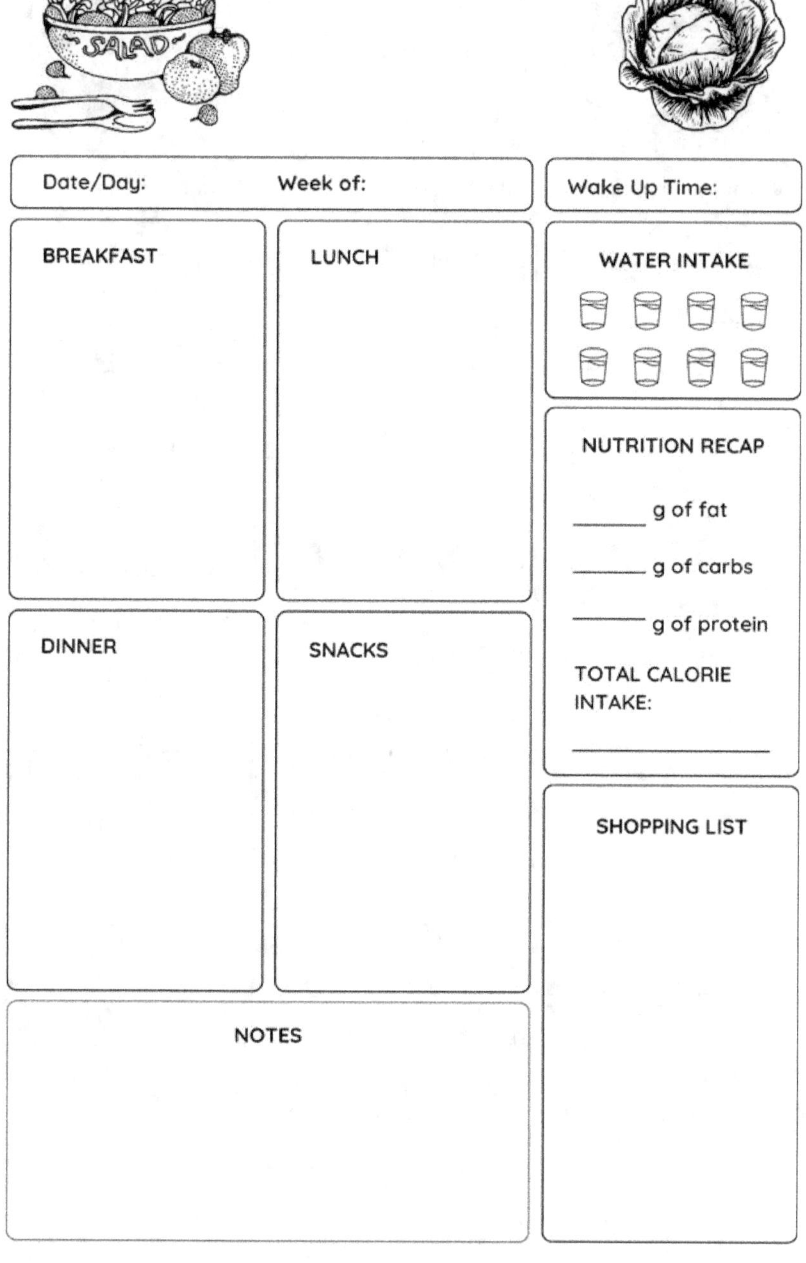

| Date/Day: | Week of: | Wake Up Time: |

BREAKFAST

LUNCH

WATER INTAKE

NUTRITION RECAP

________ g of fat

________ g of carbs

________ g of protein

TOTAL CALORIE INTAKE:

DINNER

SNACKS

SHOPPING LIST

NOTES

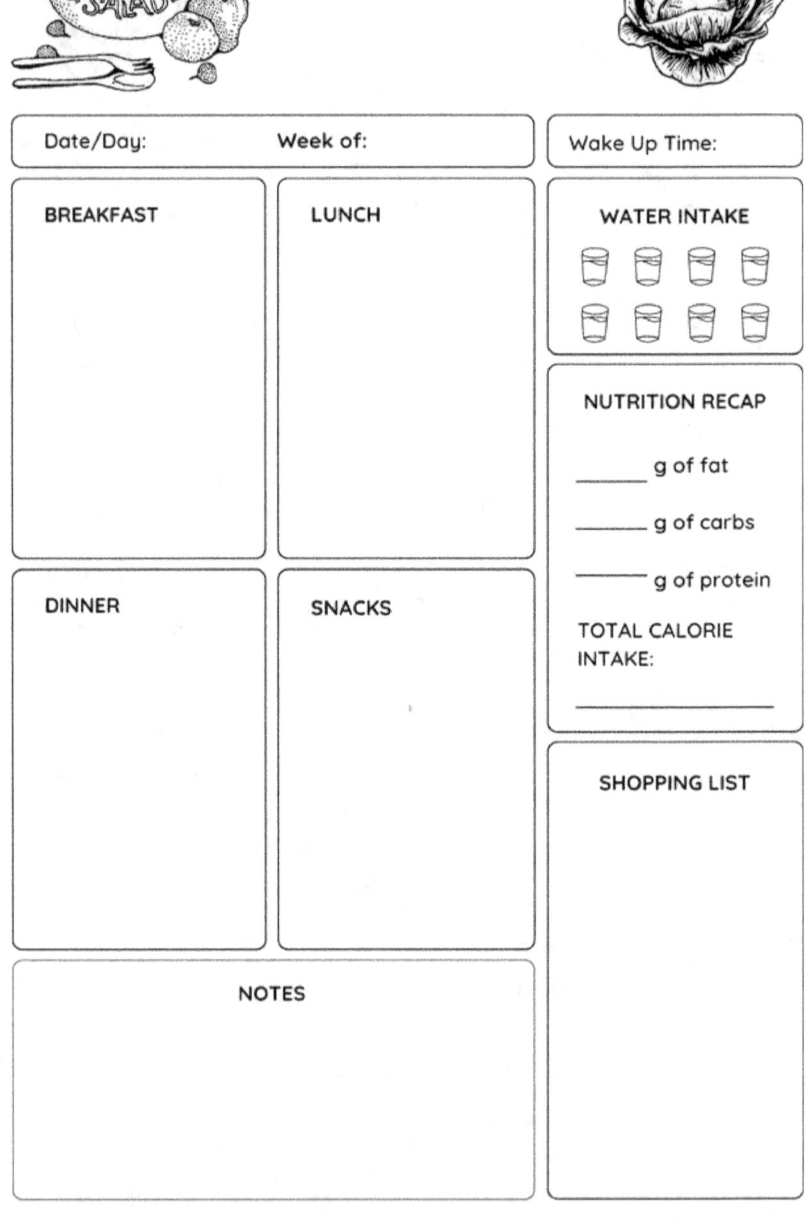

Date/Day: Week of:

Wake Up Time:

BREAKFAST

LUNCH

WATER INTAKE

NUTRITION RECAP

_______ g of fat

_______ g of carbs

_______ g of protein

TOTAL CALORIE INTAKE:

DINNER

SNACKS

SHOPPING LIST

NOTES

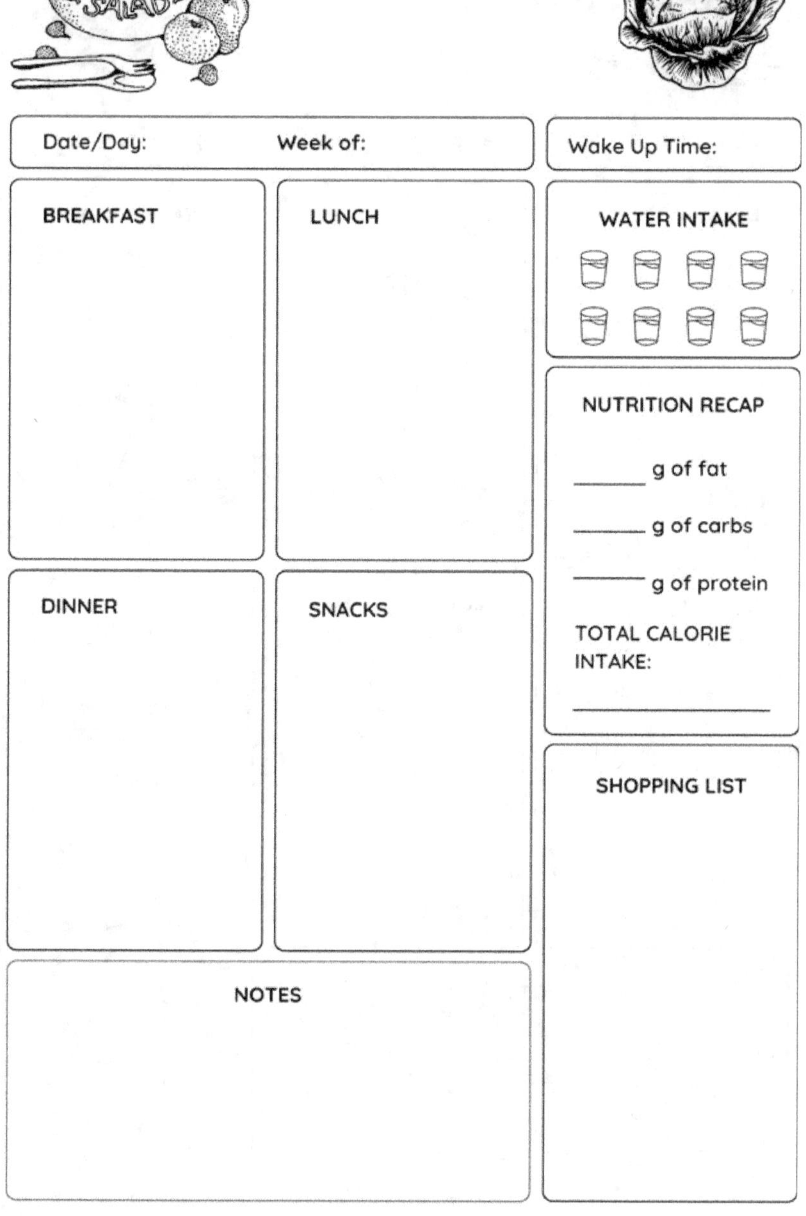

Date/Day:
Week of:
Wake Up Time:
BREAKFAST
LUNCH
WATER INTAKE
DINNER
SNACKS
NUTRITION RECAP
_______ g of fat
_______ g of carbs
_______ g of protein
TOTAL CALORIE INTAKE:
SHOPPING LIST
NOTES

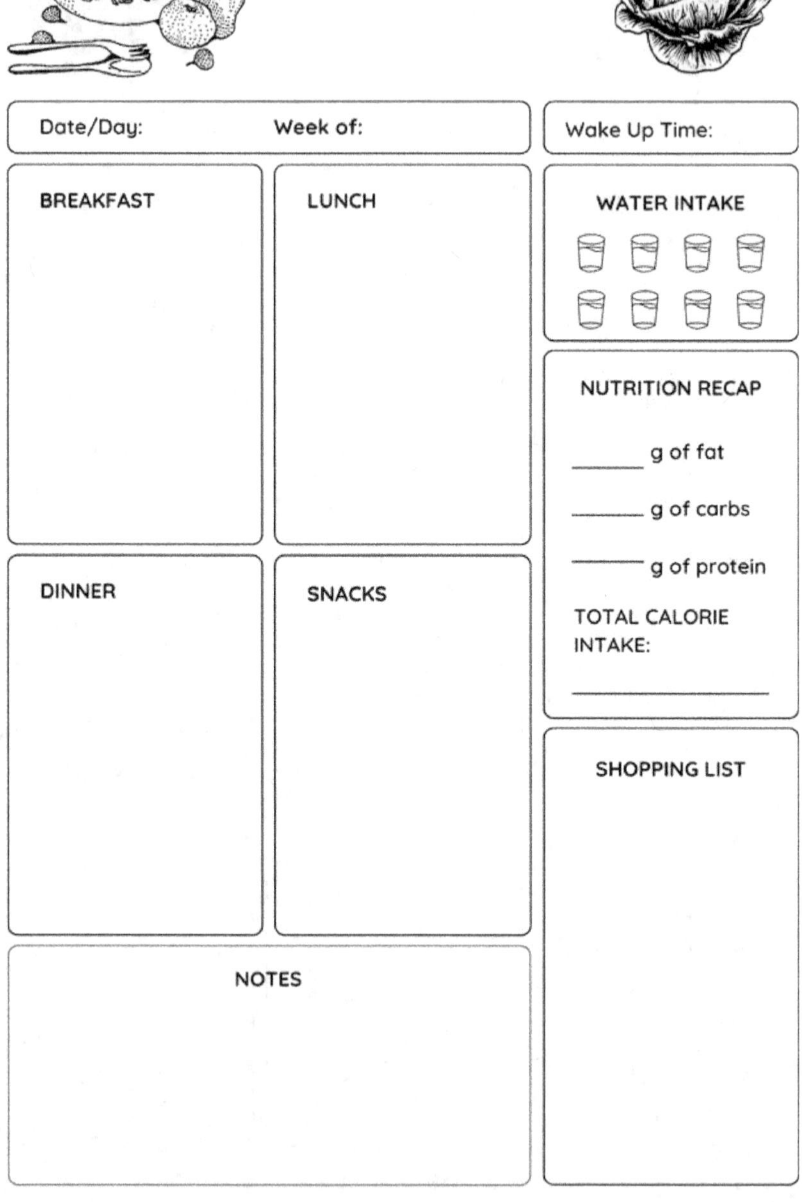

| Date/Day: | Week of: | Wake Up Time: |

BREAKFAST

LUNCH

WATER INTAKE

NUTRITION RECAP

_______ g of fat

_______ g of carbs

_______ g of protein

TOTAL CALORIE INTAKE:

____

DINNER

SNACKS

SHOPPING LIST

NOTES

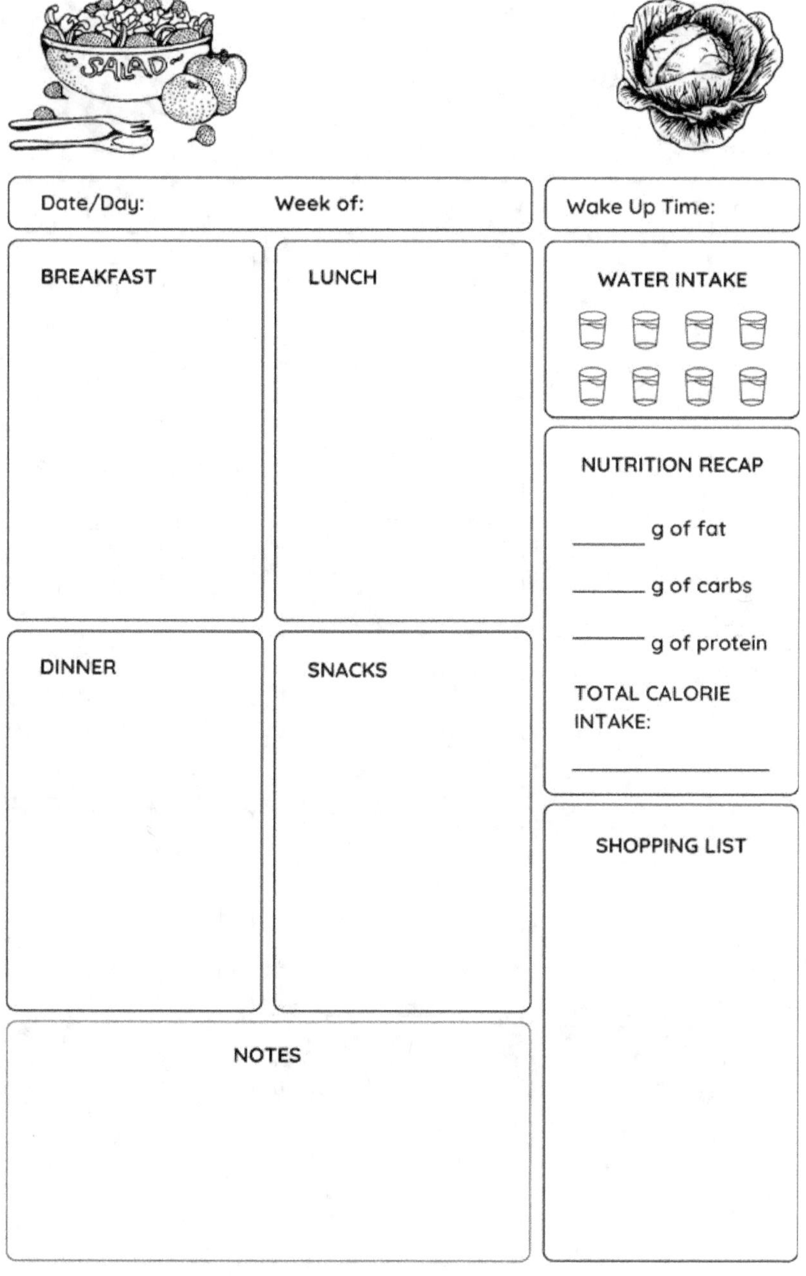
Date/Day:
Week of:
Wake Up Time:
BREAKFAST
LUNCH
WATER INTAKE
NUTRITION RECAP
_______ g of fat
_______ g of carbs
_______ g of protein
TOTAL CALORIE INTAKE:
DINNER
SNACKS
SHOPPING LIST
NOTES

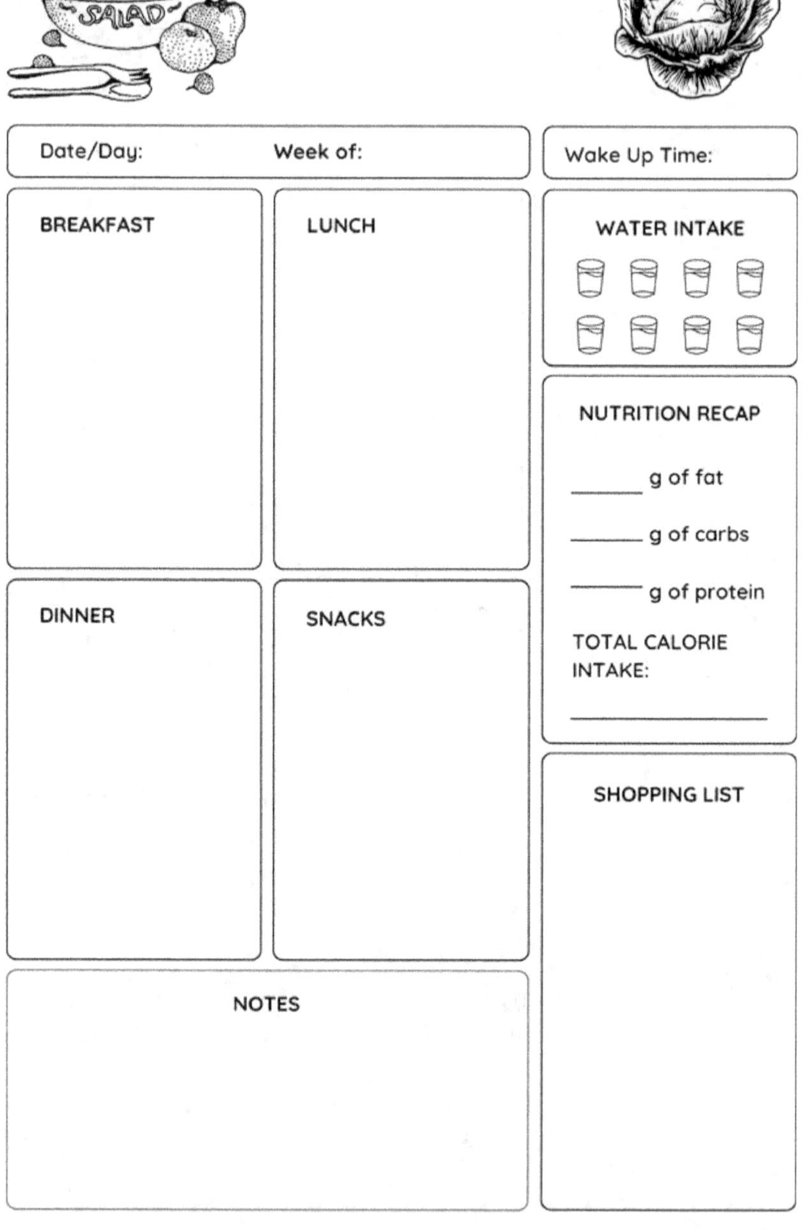

Date/Day: Week of:
Wake Up Time:
BREAKFAST
LUNCH
WATER INTAKE
NUTRITION RECAP
_______ g of fat
_______ g of carbs
_______ g of protein
TOTAL CALORIE INTAKE:
____
DINNER
SNACKS
SHOPPING LIST
NOTES

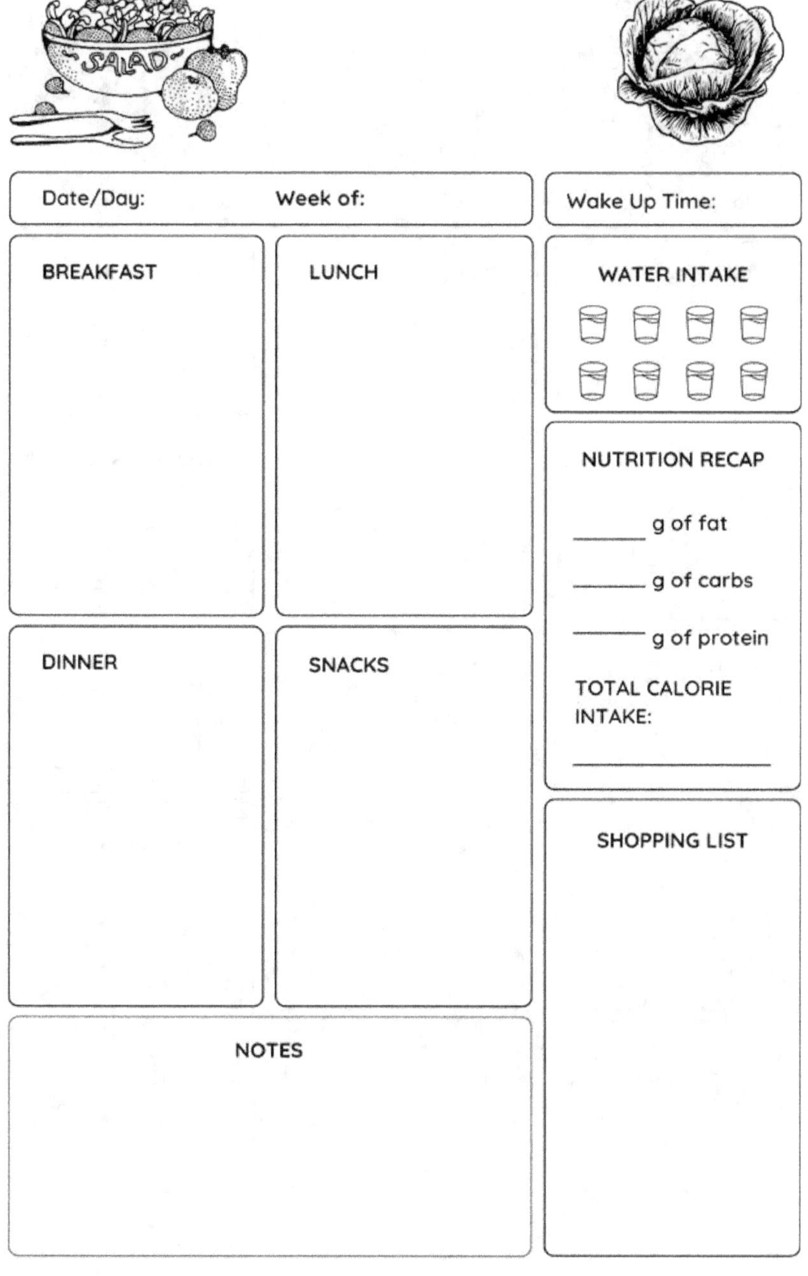

Date/Day:
Week of:
Wake Up Time:
BREAKFAST
LUNCH
WATER INTAKE
NUTRITION RECAP
_______ g of fat
_______ g of carbs
_______ g of protein
TOTAL CALORIE INTAKE:
DINNER
SNACKS
SHOPPING LIST
NOTES

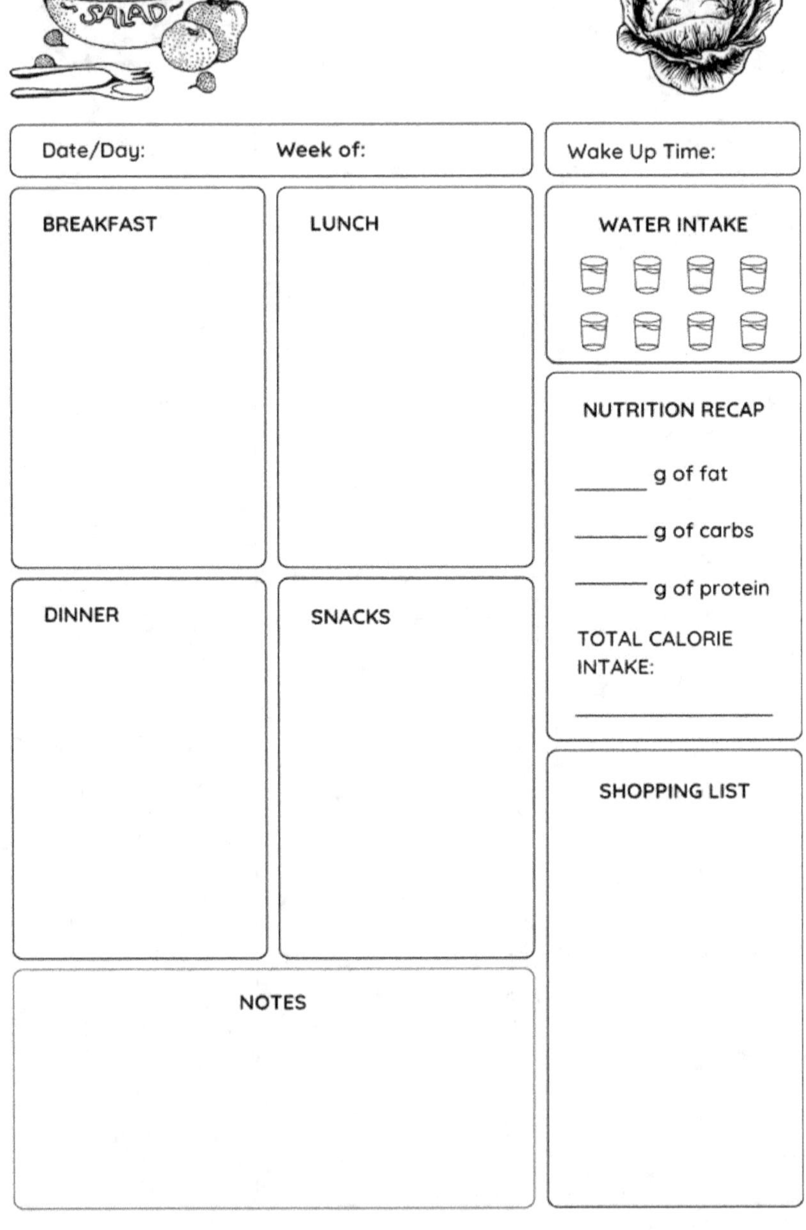
Date/Day:
Week of:
Wake Up Time:
BREAKFAST
LUNCH
WATER INTAKE
NUTRITION RECAP
_______ g of fat
_______ g of carbs
_______ g of protein
TOTAL CALORIE
INTAKE:
DINNER
SNACKS
SHOPPING LIST
NOTES

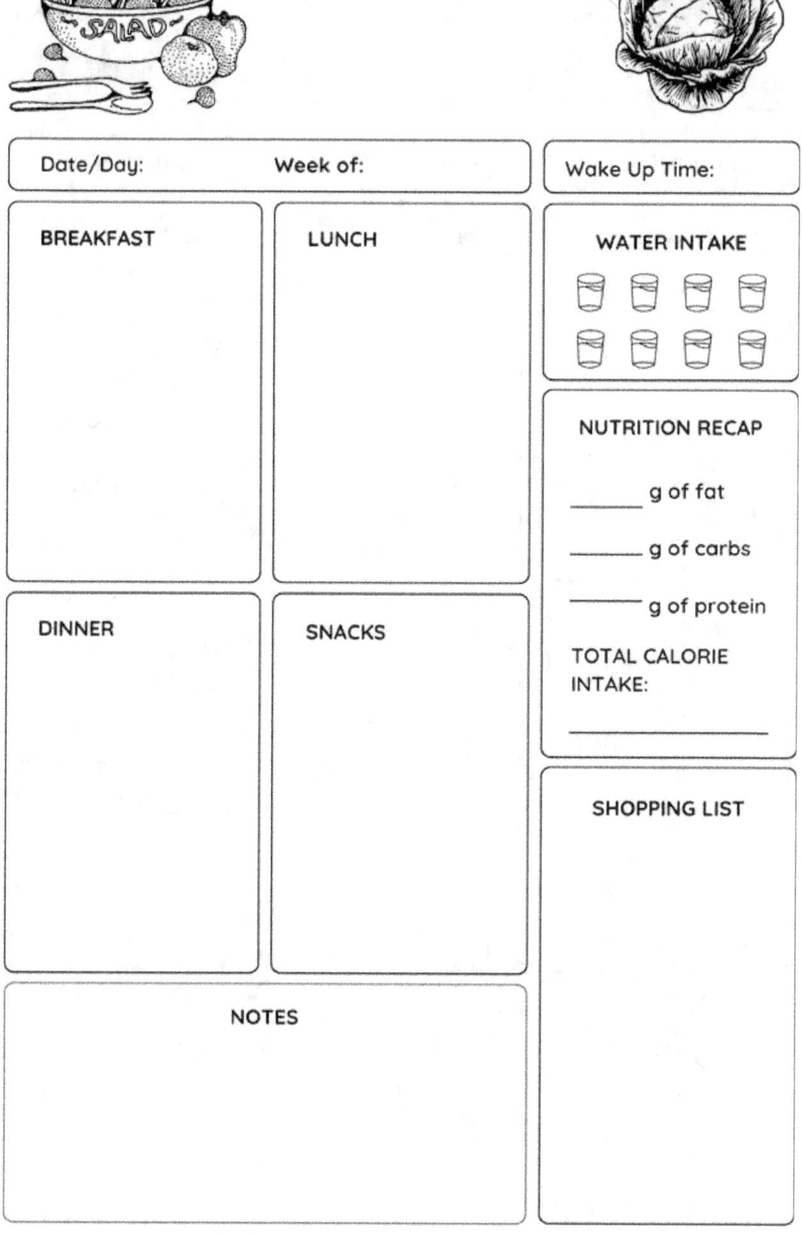

| Date/Day: | Week of: | Wake Up Time: |

BREAKFAST

LUNCH

WATER INTAKE

NUTRITION RECAP

_______ g of fat

_______ g of carbs

_______ g of protein

TOTAL CALORIE INTAKE:

DINNER

SNACKS

SHOPPING LIST

NOTES

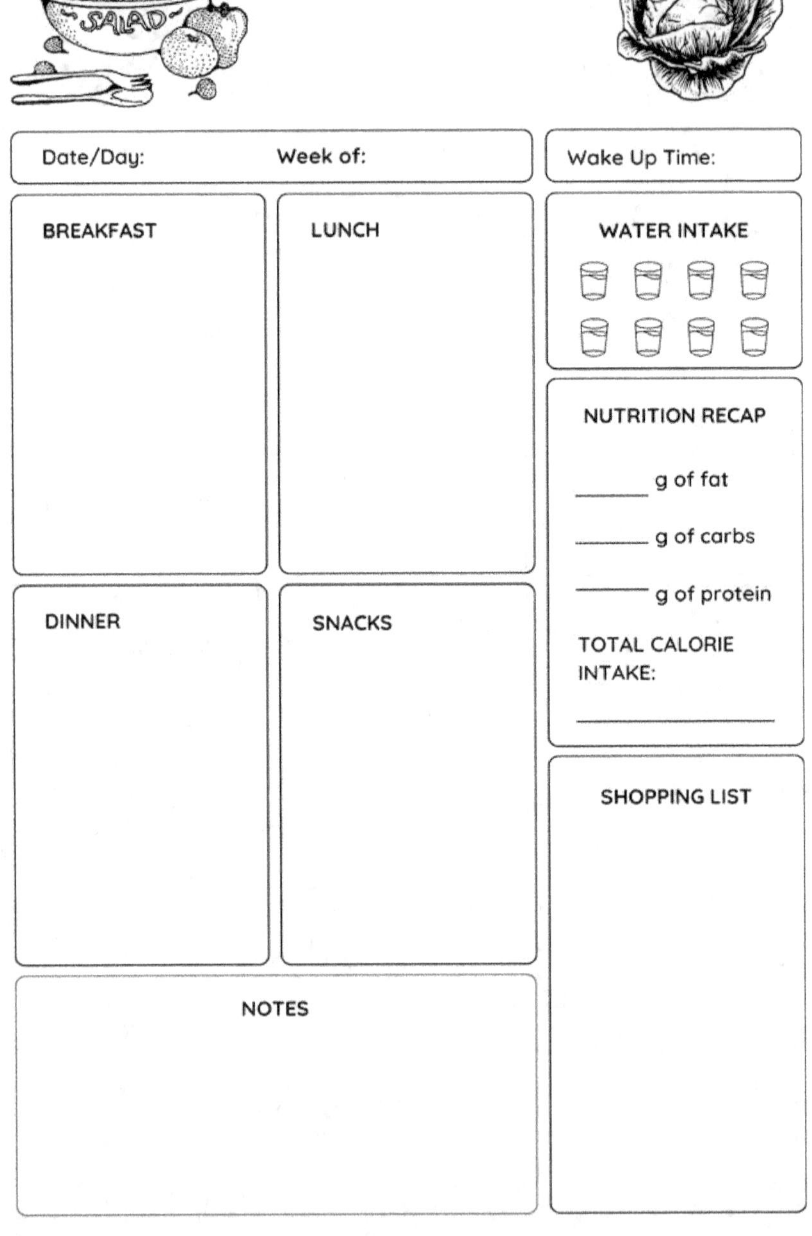

| Date/Day: | Week of: | Wake Up Time: |

BREAKFAST

LUNCH

WATER INTAKE

NUTRITION RECAP

_______ g of fat

_______ g of carbs

_______ g of protein

TOTAL CALORIE INTAKE:

DINNER

SNACKS

SHOPPING LIST

NOTES

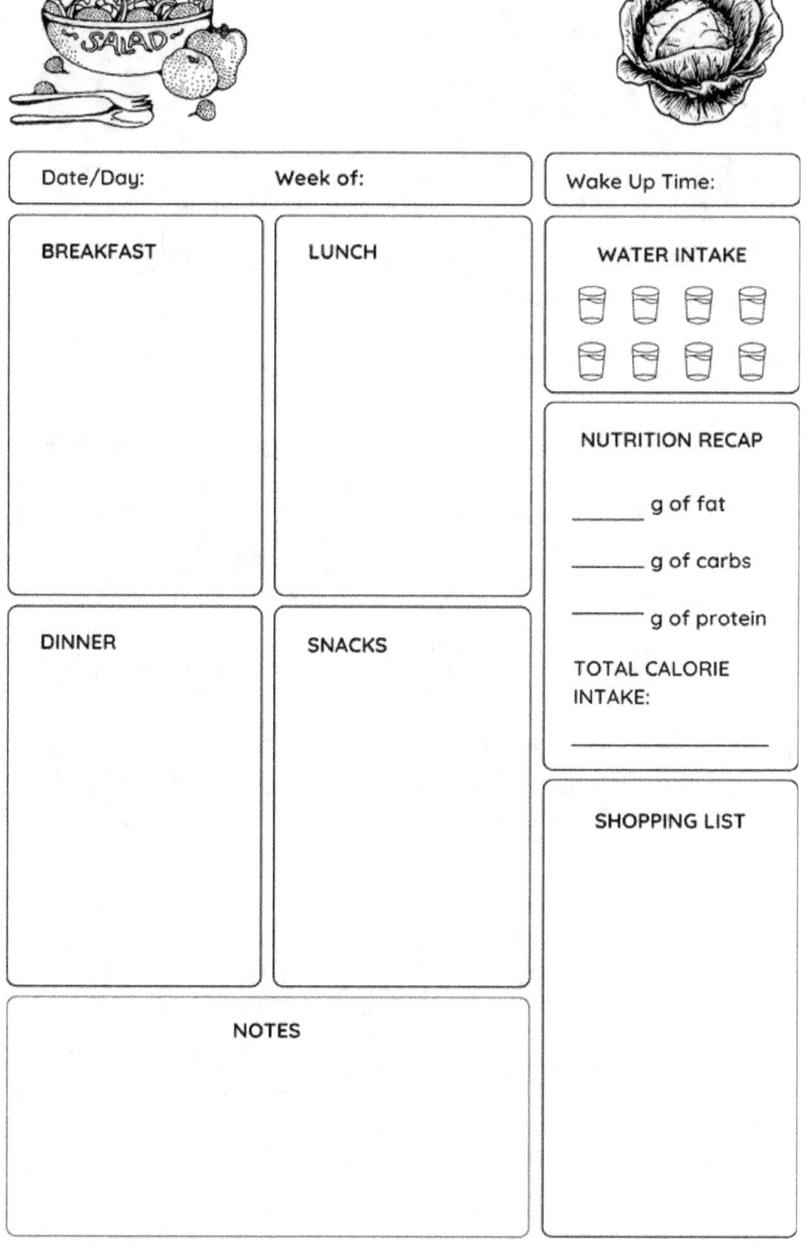

Date/Day:	Week of:	Wake Up Time:

BREAKFAST

LUNCH

WATER INTAKE

NUTRITION RECAP

_______ g of fat

_______ g of carbs

_______ g of protein

TOTAL CALORIE INTAKE:

____

DINNER

SNACKS

SHOPPING LIST

NOTES

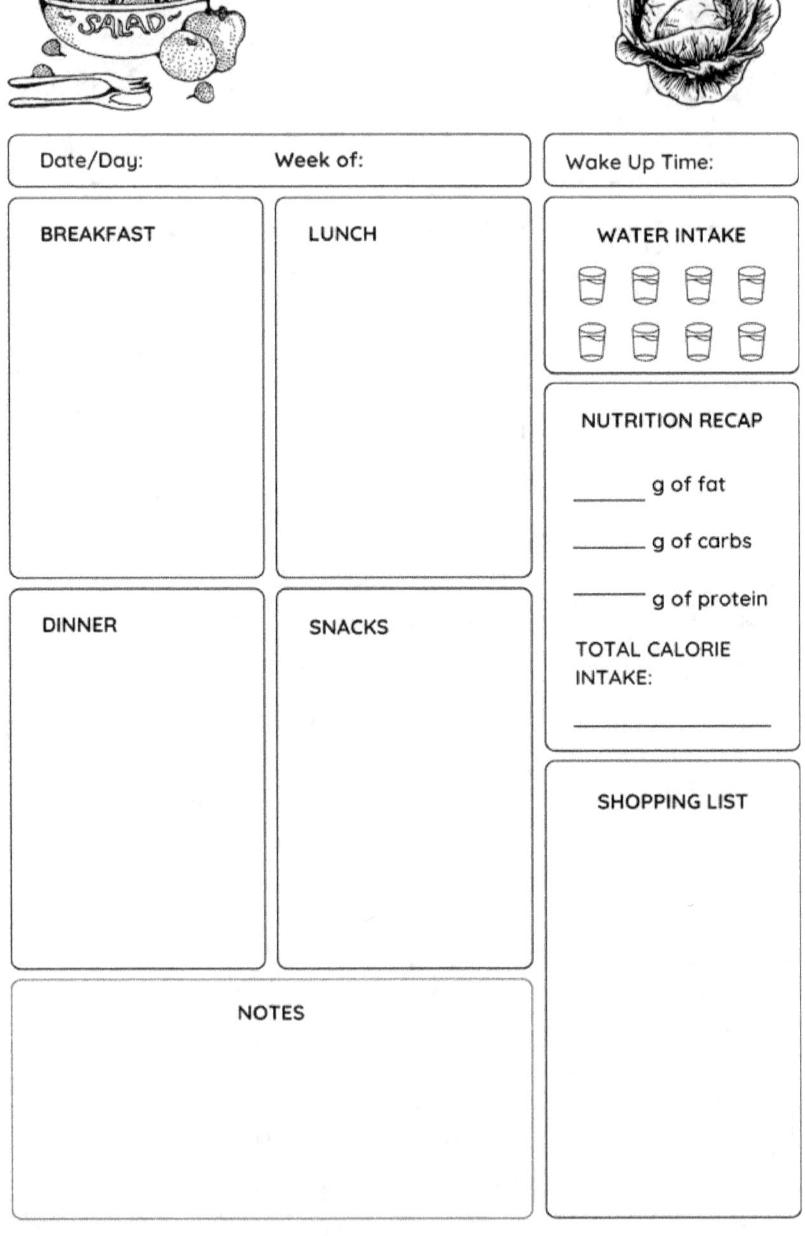

Date/Day: Week of:

Wake Up Time:

BREAKFAST

LUNCH

WATER INTAKE

NUTRITION RECAP

_______ g of fat

_______ g of carbs

_______ g of protein

TOTAL CALORIE INTAKE:

____

DINNER

SNACKS

SHOPPING LIST

NOTES

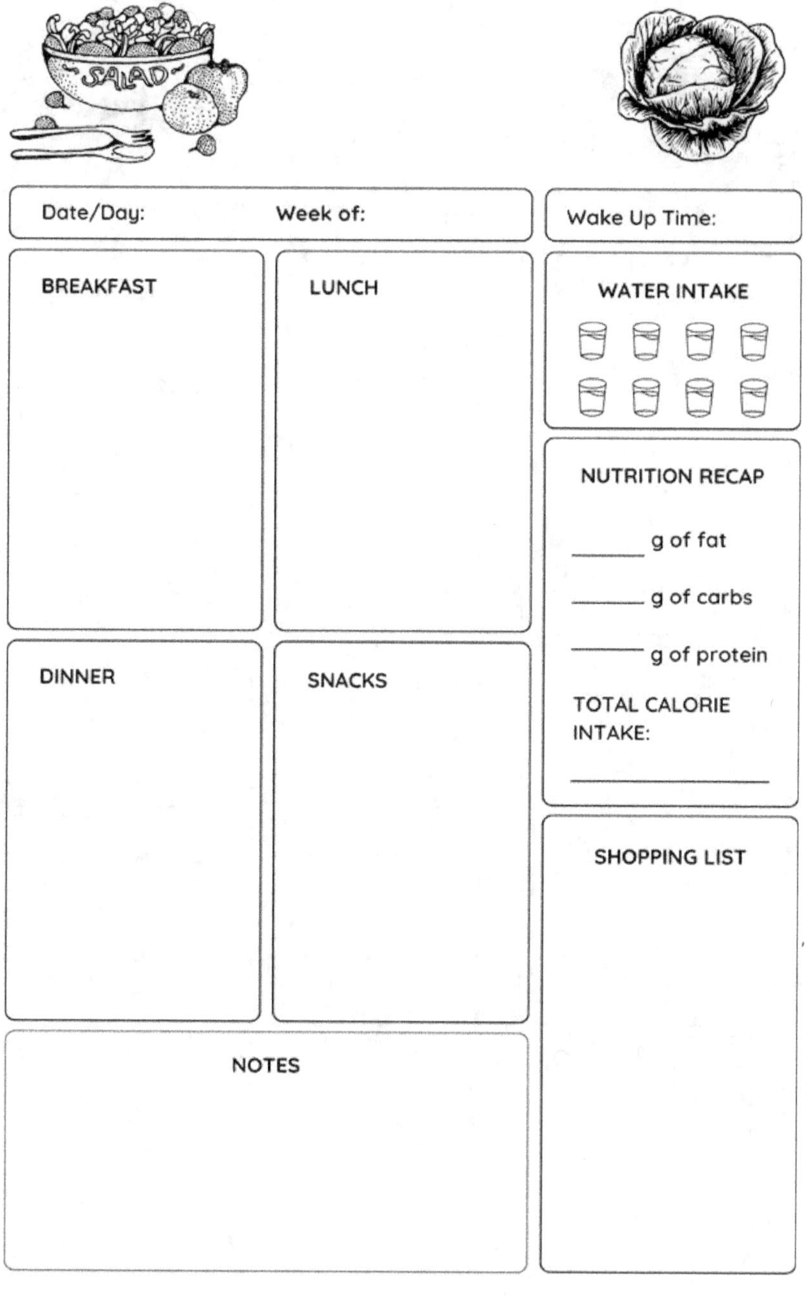

Date/Day: Week of:

Wake Up Time:

BREAKFAST

LUNCH

WATER INTAKE

NUTRITION RECAP

_________ g of fat

_________ g of carbs

_________ g of protein

TOTAL CALORIE INTAKE:

____

DINNER

SNACKS

SHOPPING LIST

NOTES

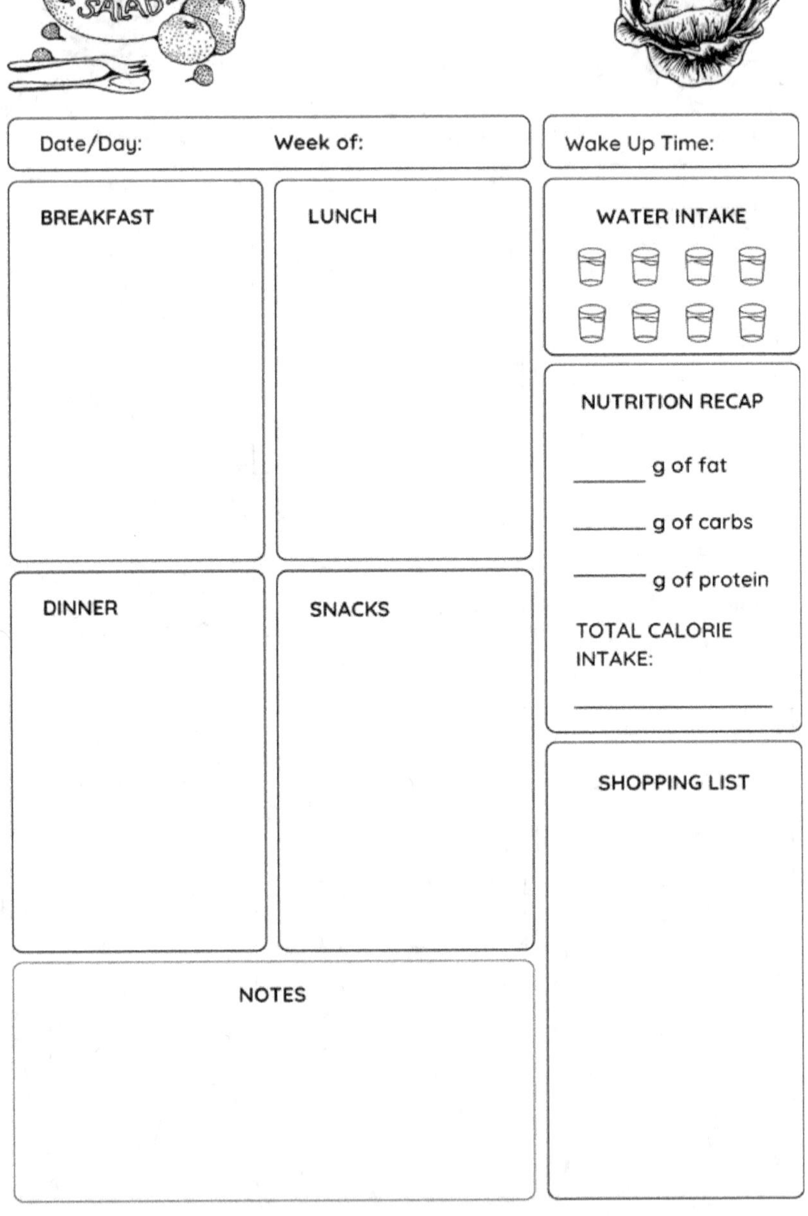
Date/Day: Week of:
Wake Up Time:
BREAKFAST
LUNCH
WATER INTAKE
NUTRITION RECAP
_______ g of fat
_______ g of carbs
_______ g of protein
TOTAL CALORIE
INTAKE:
DINNER
SNACKS
SHOPPING LIST
NOTES

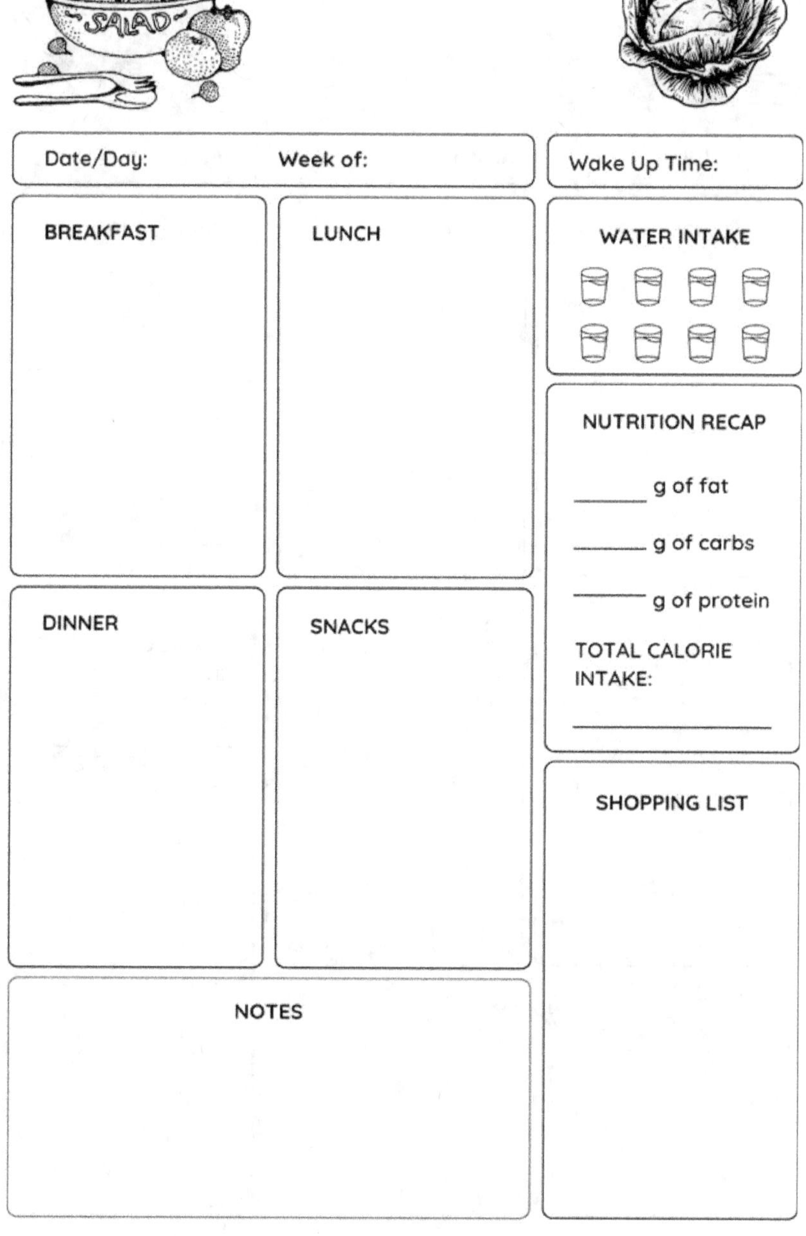

Date/Day: Week of:

Wake Up Time:

BREAKFAST

LUNCH

WATER INTAKE

NUTRITION RECAP

_______ g of fat

_______ g of carbs

_______ g of protein

TOTAL CALORIE INTAKE:

____

DINNER

SNACKS

SHOPPING LIST

NOTES

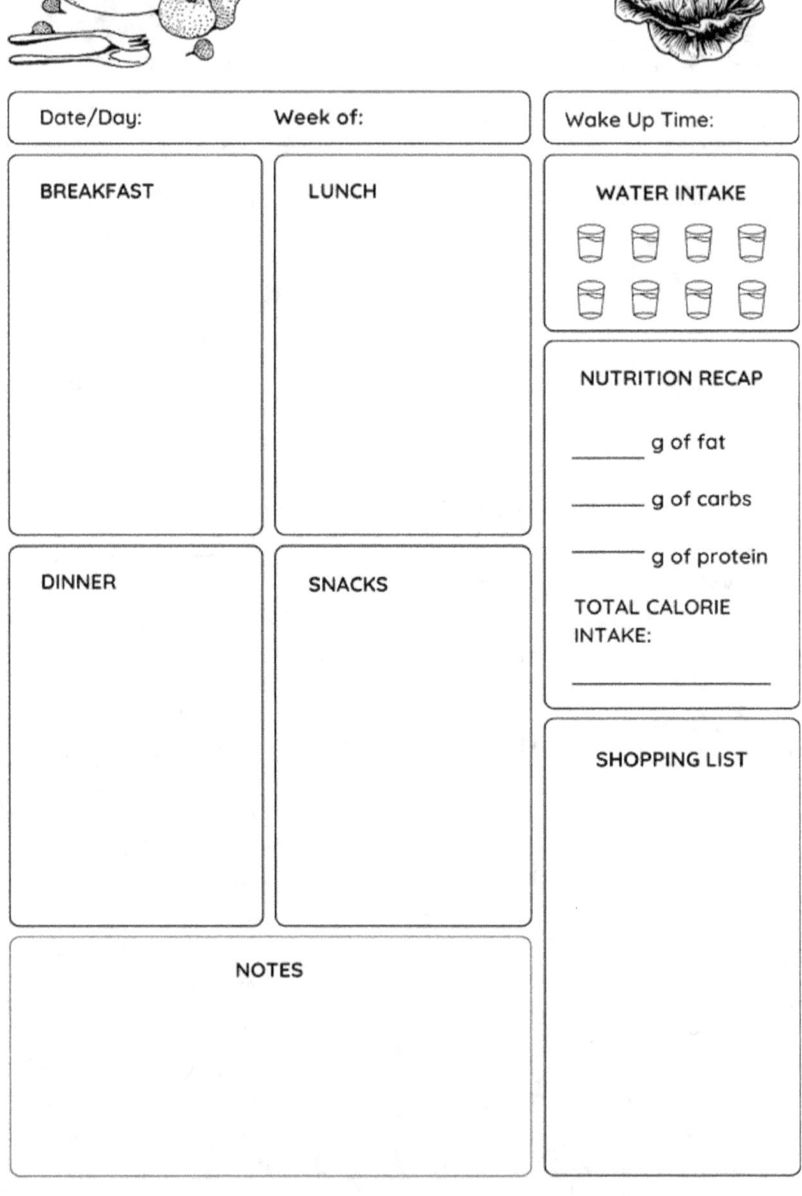

Date/Day: Week of:

Wake Up Time:

BREAKFAST

LUNCH

WATER INTAKE

NUTRITION RECAP

_______ g of fat

_______ g of carbs

_______ g of protein

TOTAL CALORIE INTAKE:

____

DINNER

SNACKS

SHOPPING LIST

NOTES

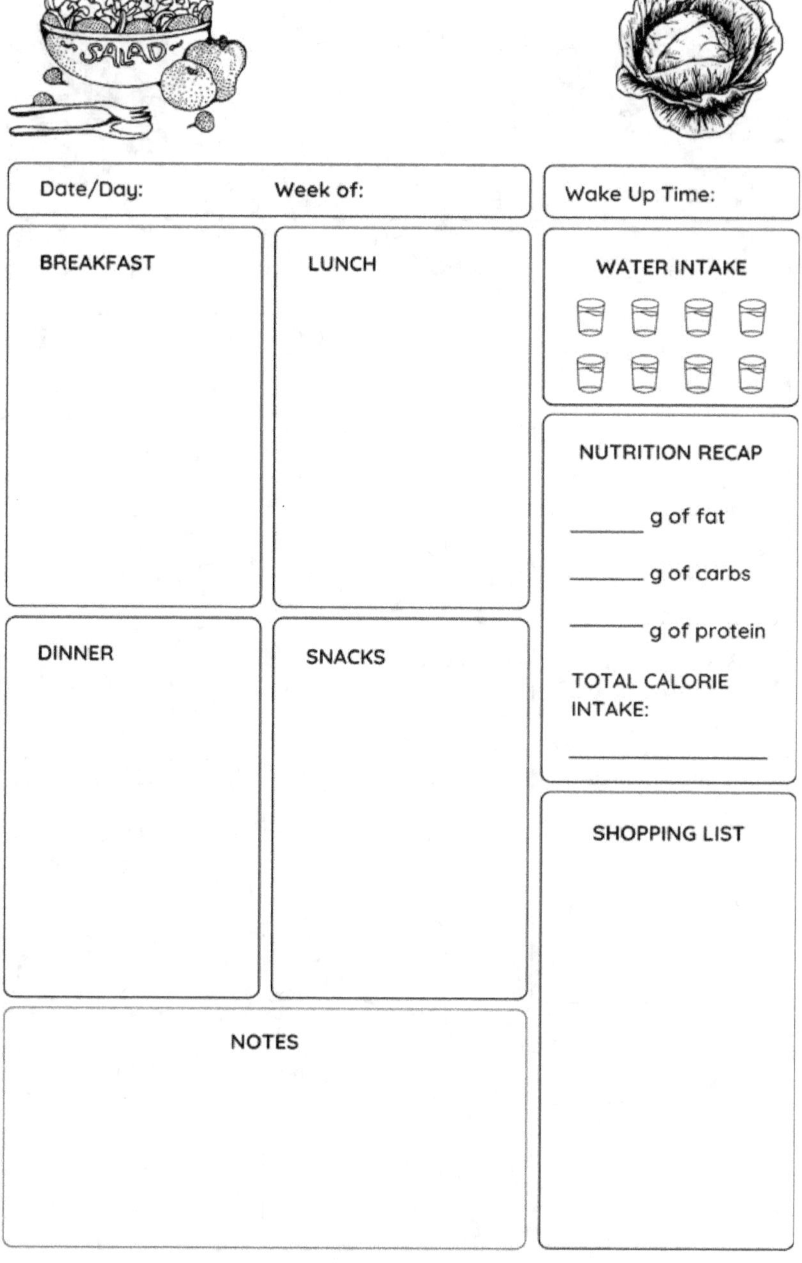

Date/Day: Week of:

Wake Up Time:

BREAKFAST

LUNCH

WATER INTAKE

NUTRITION RECAP

_______ g of fat

_______ g of carbs

_______ g of protein

TOTAL CALORIE
INTAKE:

____

DINNER

SNACKS

SHOPPING LIST

NOTES

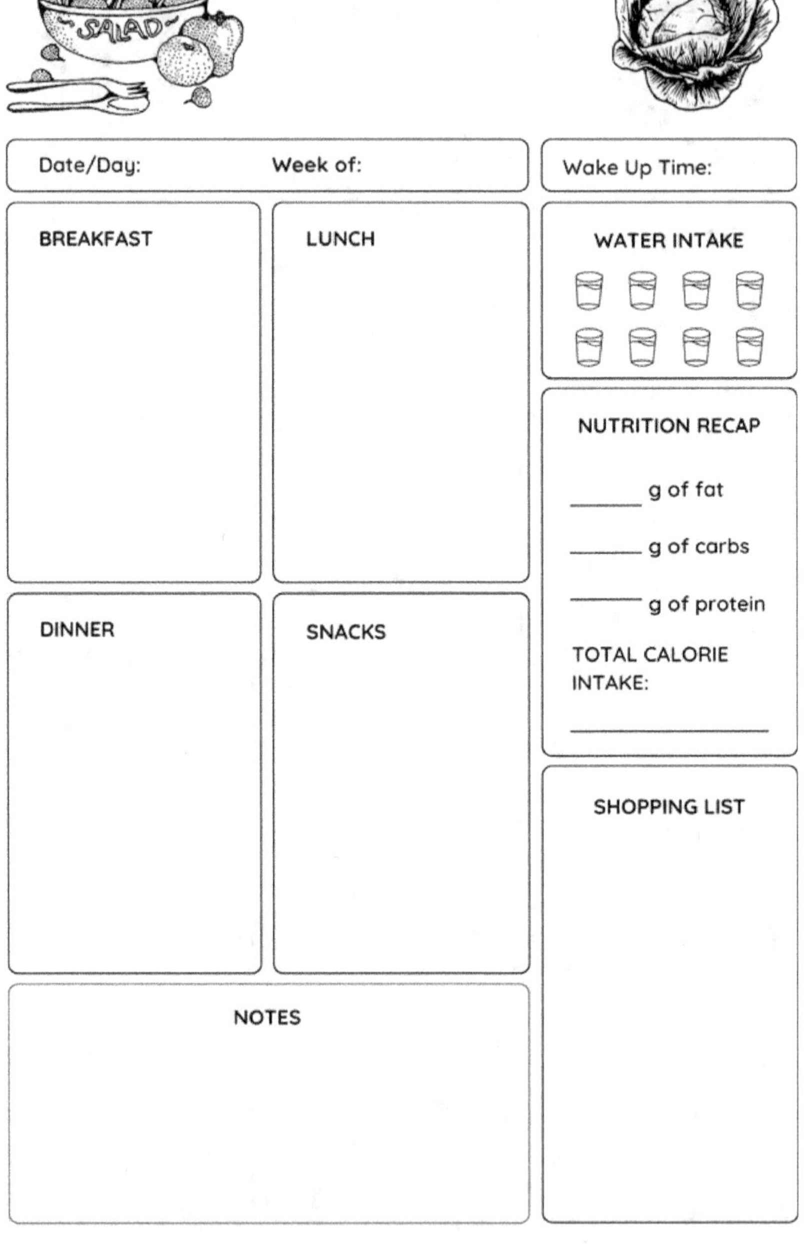

Date/Day: Week of:

Wake Up Time:

BREAKFAST

LUNCH

WATER INTAKE

NUTRITION RECAP

_______ g of fat

_______ g of carbs

_______ g of protein

TOTAL CALORIE
INTAKE:
____

DINNER

SNACKS

SHOPPING LIST

NOTES

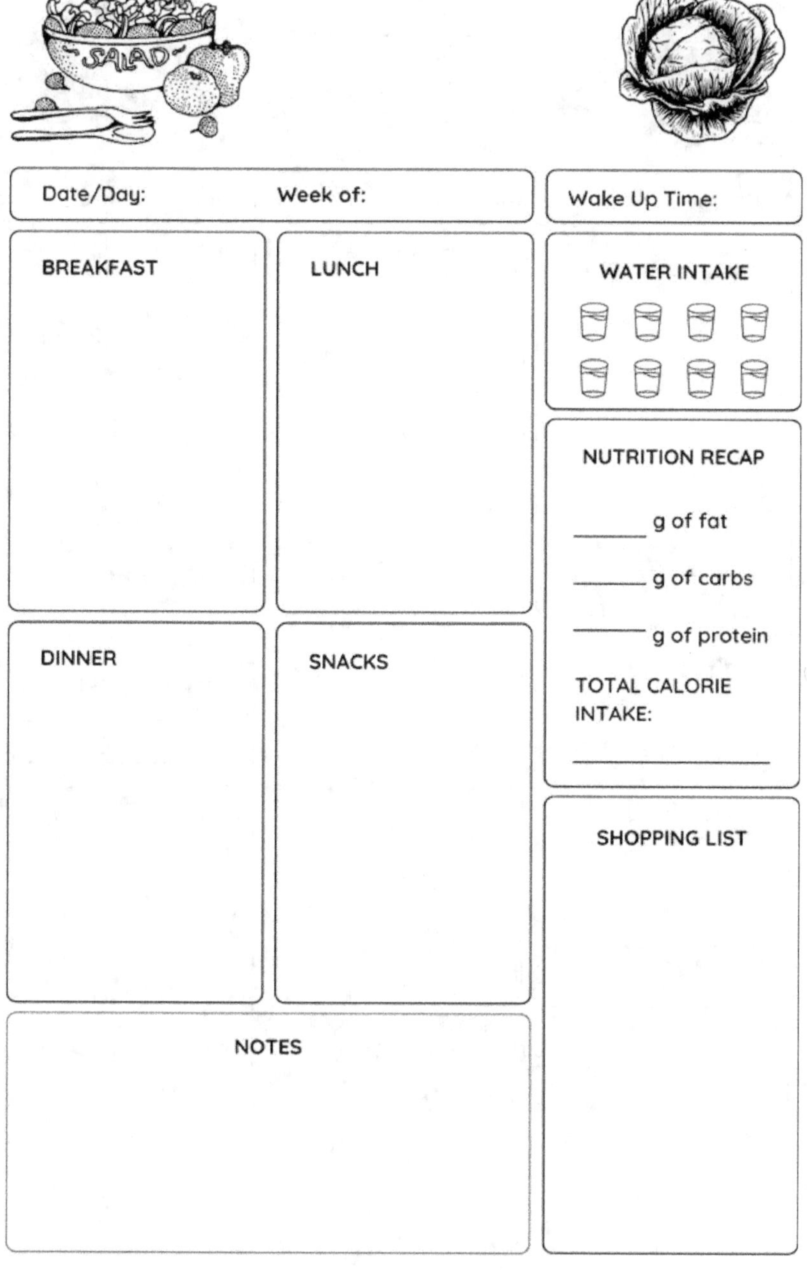

| Date/Day: | Week of: | Wake Up Time: |

BREAKFAST

LUNCH

WATER INTAKE

NUTRITION RECAP

_______ g of fat

_______ g of carbs

_______ g of protein

TOTAL CALORIE INTAKE:

____

DINNER

SNACKS

SHOPPING LIST

NOTES

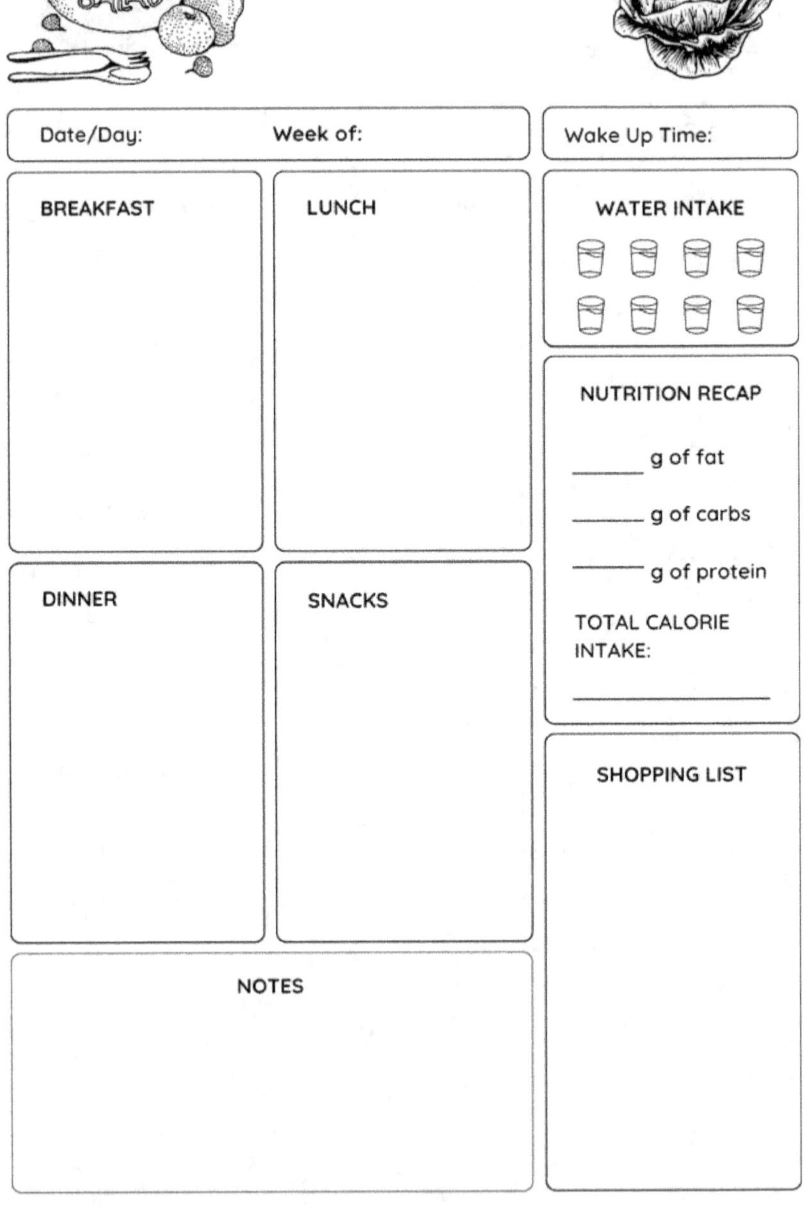

| Date/Day: | Week of: | Wake Up Time: |

BREAKFAST

LUNCH

WATER INTAKE

NUTRITION RECAP

______ g of fat

______ g of carbs

______ g of protein

TOTAL CALORIE INTAKE:

____

DINNER

SNACKS

SHOPPING LIST

NOTES

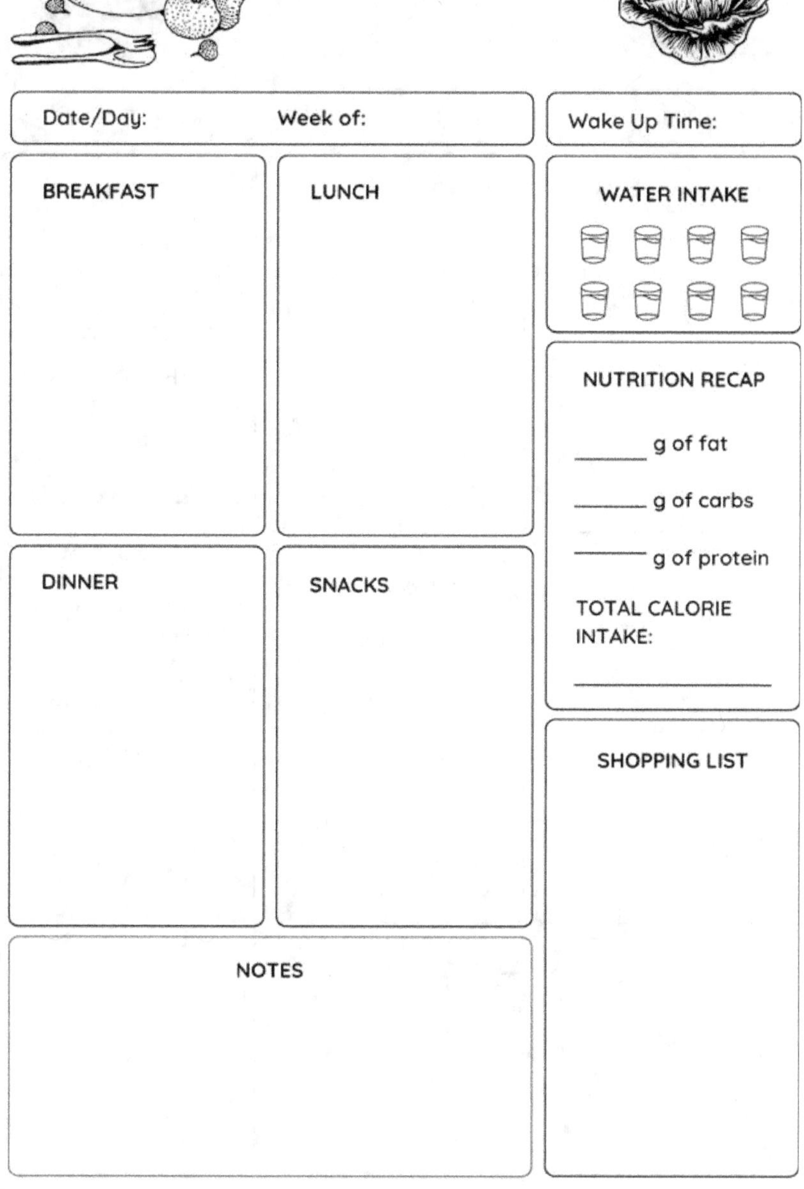

Date/Day: Week of:

Wake Up Time:

BREAKFAST

LUNCH

WATER INTAKE

DINNER

SNACKS

NUTRITION RECAP

_________ g of fat

_________ g of carbs

_________ g of protein

TOTAL CALORIE INTAKE:

____

SHOPPING LIST

NOTES

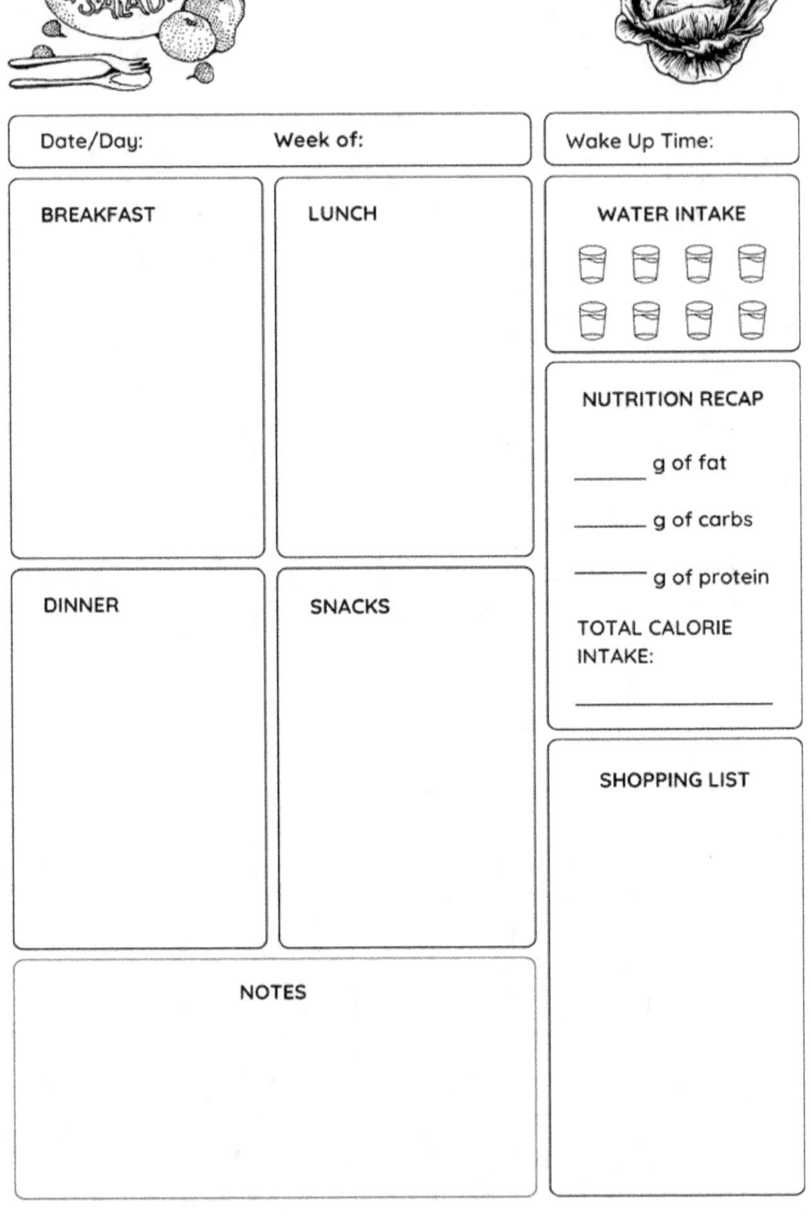

| Date/Day: | Week of: | Wake Up Time: |

BREAKFAST

LUNCH

WATER INTAKE

NUTRITION RECAP

_________ g of fat

_________ g of carbs

_________ g of protein

TOTAL CALORIE INTAKE:

DINNER

SNACKS

SHOPPING LIST

NOTES

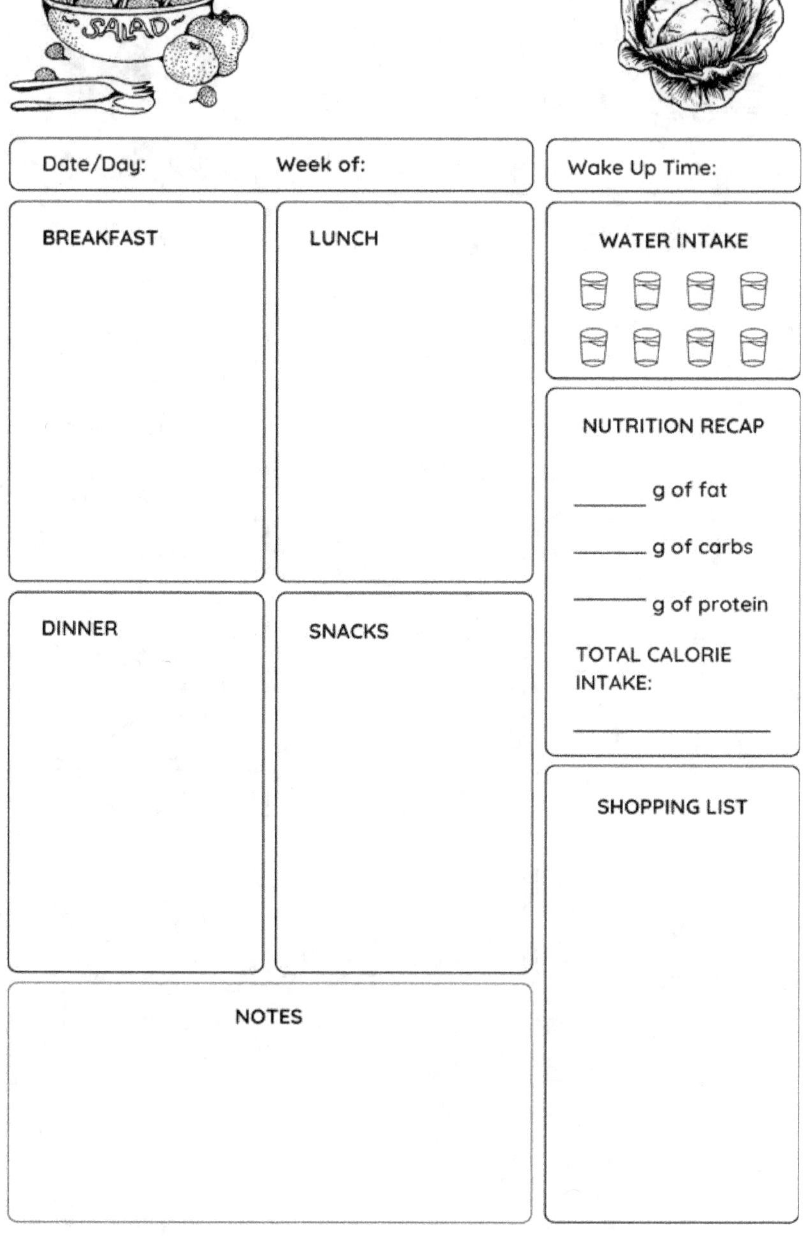

| Date/Day: | Week of: | Wake Up Time: |

BREAKFAST

LUNCH

WATER INTAKE

NUTRITION RECAP

_______ g of fat

_______ g of carbs

_______ g of protein

TOTAL CALORIE INTAKE:

DINNER

SNACKS

SHOPPING LIST

NOTES

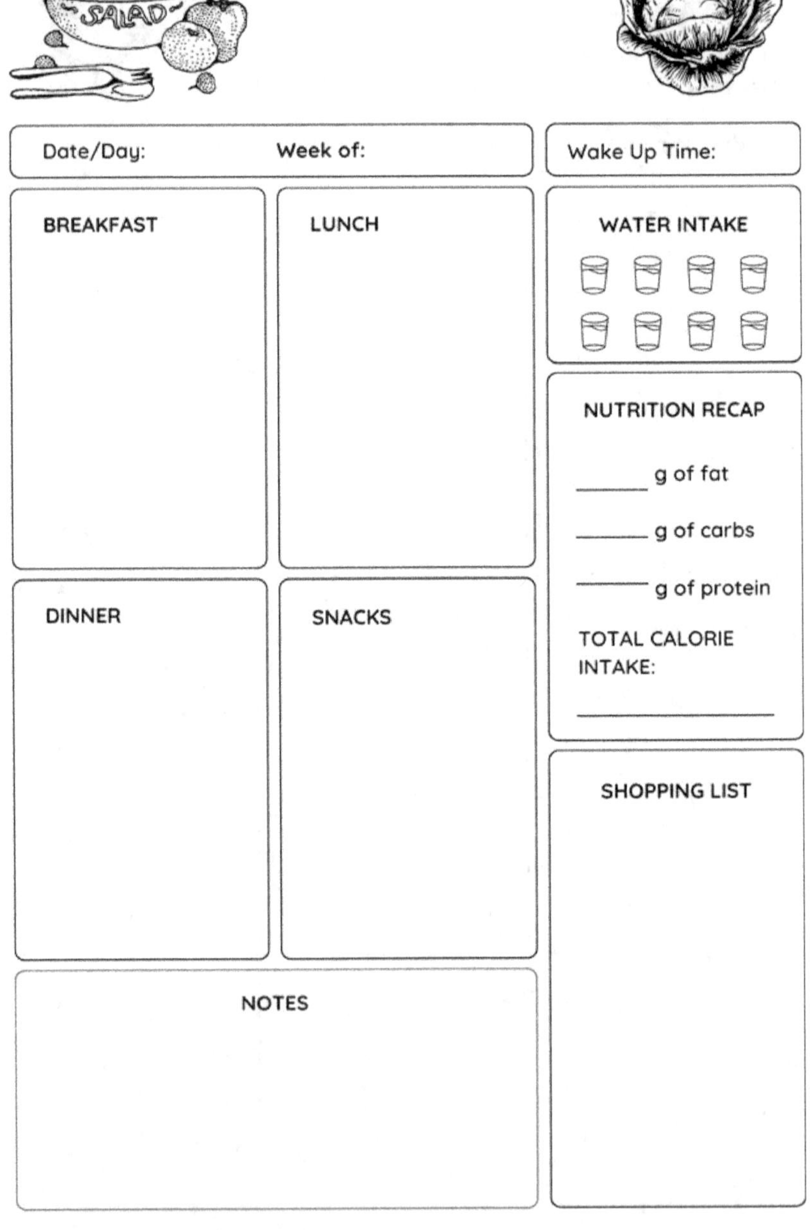

| Date/Day: | Week of: | Wake Up Time: |

BREAKFAST

LUNCH

WATER INTAKE

DINNER

SNACKS

NUTRITION RECAP

_______ g of fat

_______ g of carbs

_______ g of protein

TOTAL CALORIE INTAKE:

____

SHOPPING LIST

NOTES

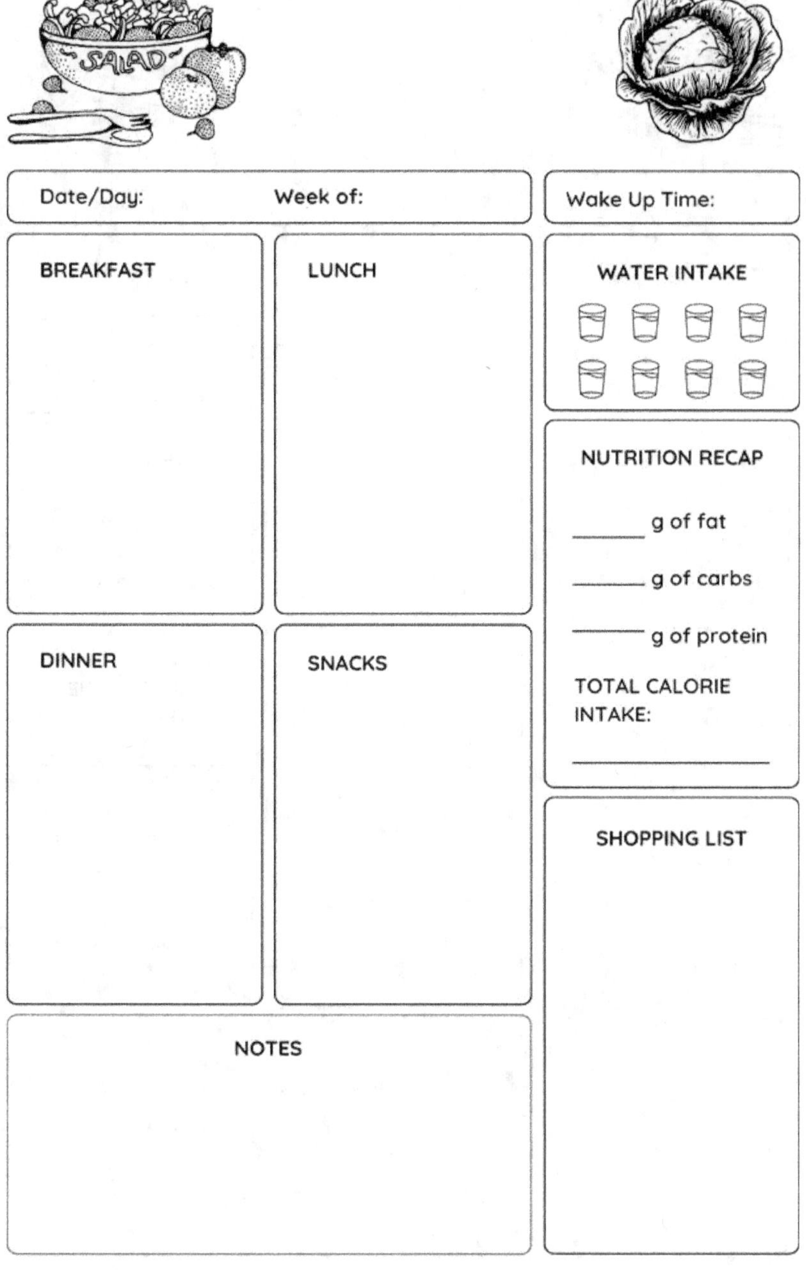

Date/Day: **Week of:**

Wake Up Time:

BREAKFAST

LUNCH

WATER INTAKE

NUTRITION RECAP

_________ g of fat

_________ g of carbs

_________ g of protein

TOTAL CALORIE INTAKE:

____

DINNER

SNACKS

SHOPPING LIST

NOTES

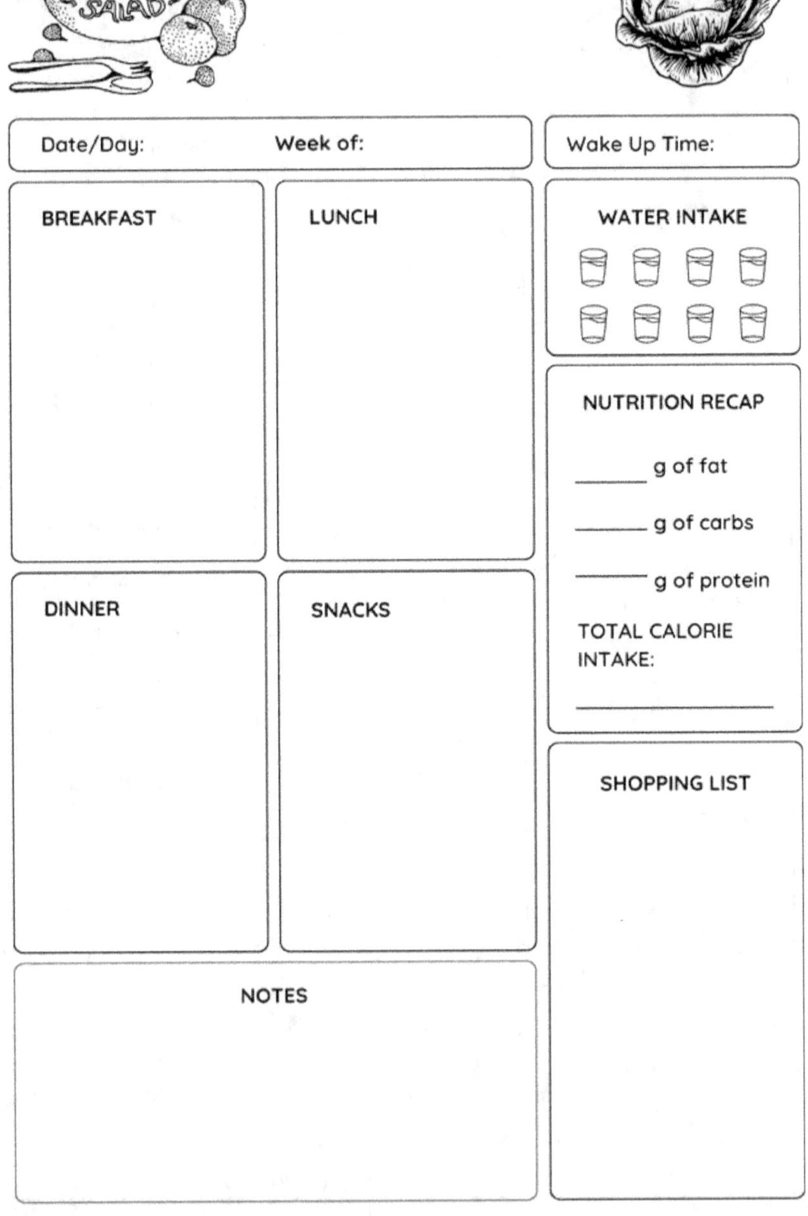

| Date/Day: | Week of: | Wake Up Time: |

BREAKFAST

LUNCH

WATER INTAKE

NUTRITION RECAP

_______ g of fat

_______ g of carbs

_______ g of protein

TOTAL CALORIE INTAKE:

____

DINNER

SNACKS

SHOPPING LIST

NOTES

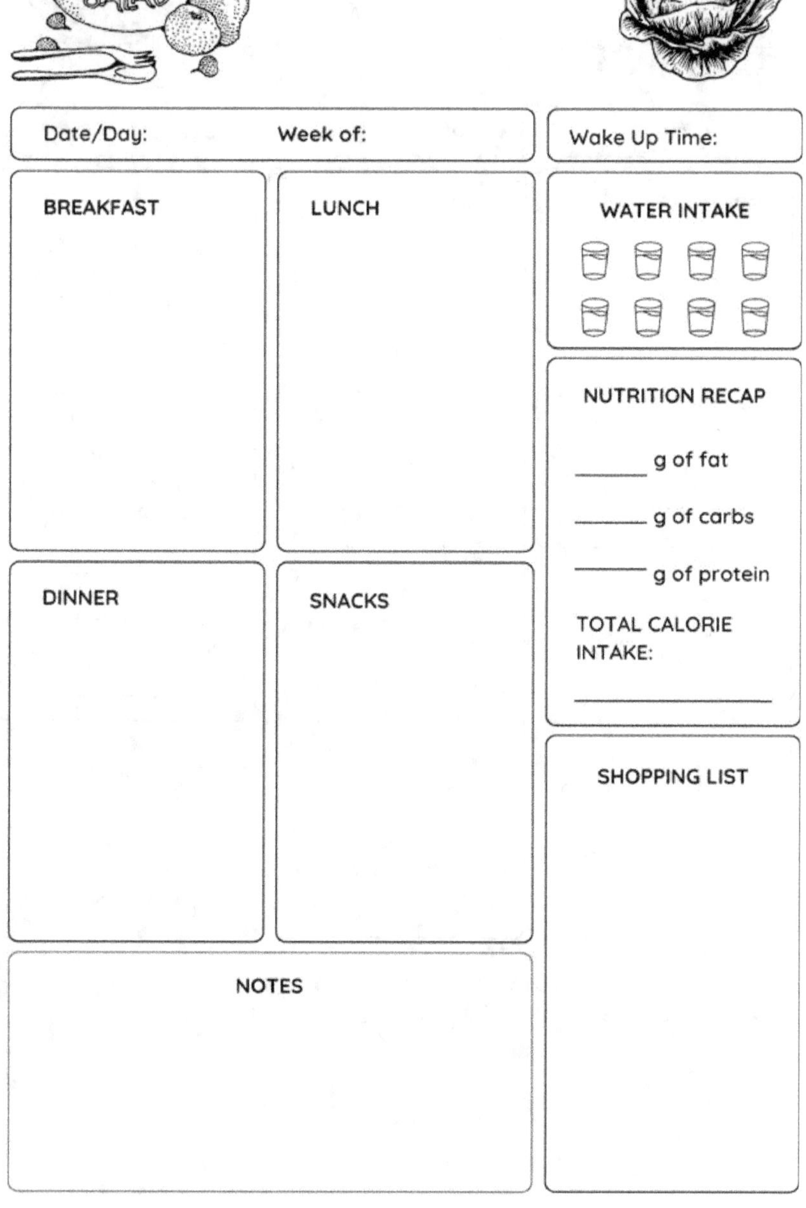

| Date/Day: | Week of: | Wake Up Time: |

BREAKFAST

LUNCH

WATER INTAKE

NUTRITION RECAP

_______ g of fat

_______ g of carbs

_______ g of protein

TOTAL CALORIE INTAKE:

____

DINNER

SNACKS

SHOPPING LIST

NOTES

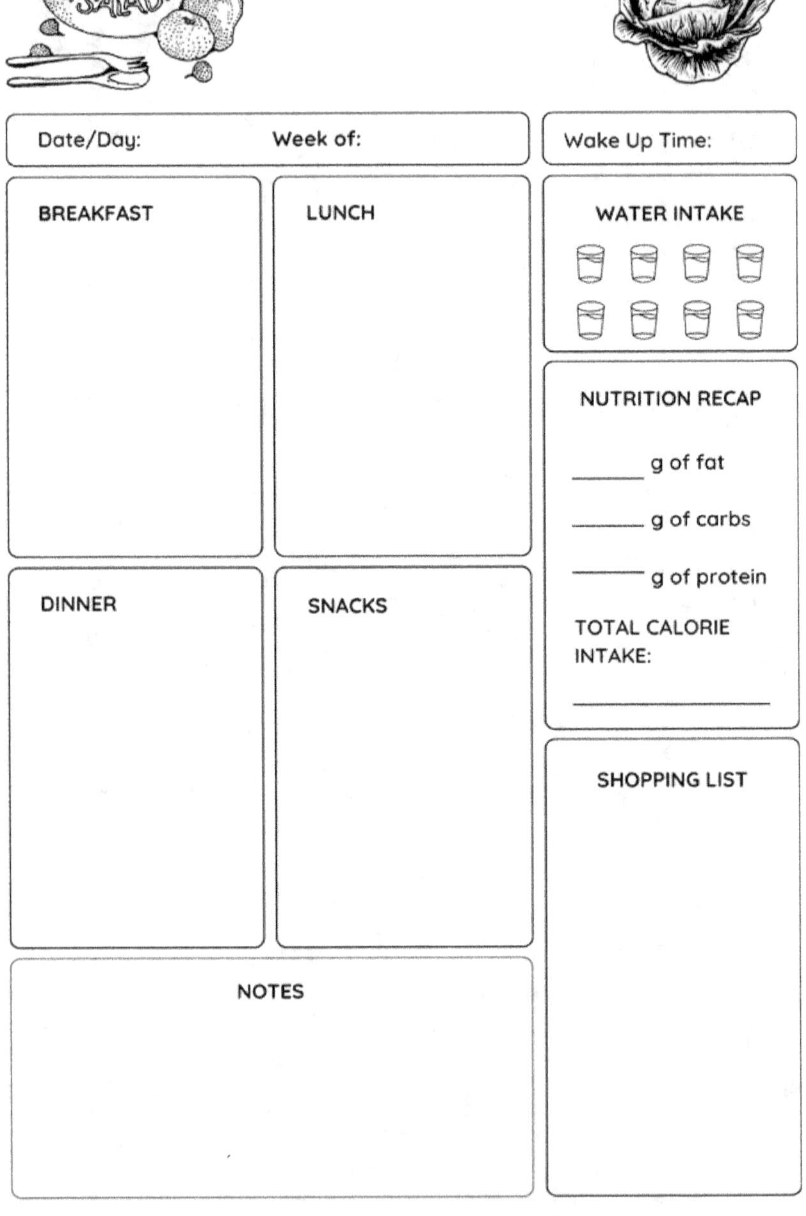

Date/Day: Week of:

Wake Up Time:

BREAKFAST

LUNCH

WATER INTAKE

NUTRITION RECAP

_______ g of fat

_______ g of carbs

_______ g of protein

TOTAL CALORIE INTAKE:

____

DINNER

SNACKS

SHOPPING LIST

NOTES

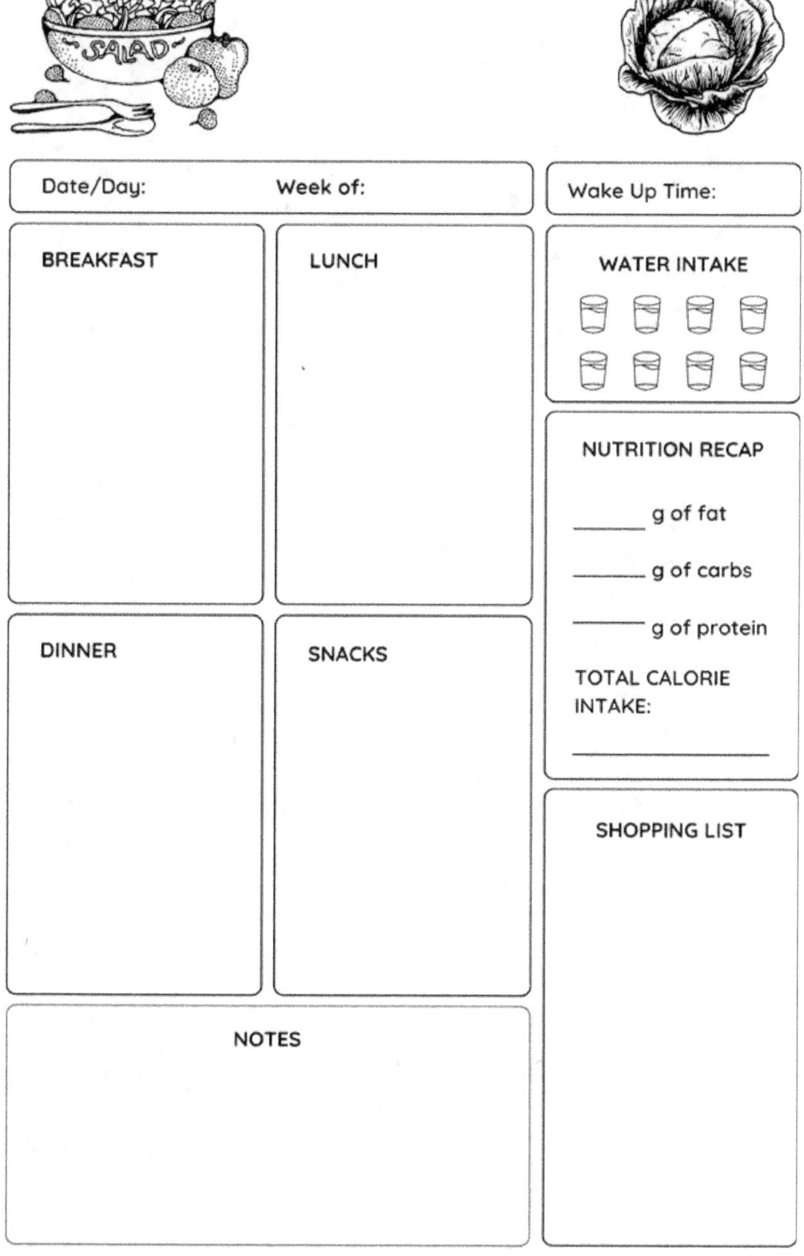

| Date/Day: | Week of: | Wake Up Time: |

BREAKFAST

LUNCH

WATER INTAKE

NUTRITION RECAP

_______ g of fat

_______ g of carbs

_______ g of protein

TOTAL CALORIE INTAKE:

____

DINNER

SNACKS

SHOPPING LIST

NOTES